CHAIR YOGA FOR SENIORS OVER 60

A 28-DAY CHALLENGE

Linette Cunley

DISCLAIMER

The information in this book is provided for educational and entertainment purposes only. Every effort has been made to present accurate, up-to-date, and reliable information. However, no warranties of any kind are expressed or implied. The author does not offer legal, financial, medical, or professional advice. Readers are strongly encouraged to consult a licensed professional before attempting any of the techniques described in this book.

HEALTH AND SAFETY NOTICE

This book is not intended to diagnose, treat, cure, or prevent any medical condition. The information provided is for educational purposes only and should not be considered medical advice. Always consult with a qualified healthcare professional before beginning any exercise program or implementing any suggestions from this book, especially if you have pre-existing conditions, injuries, or concerns about your physical or mental health. The author and publisher are not responsible for any health-related issues that may arise from the use of the information in this book.

By reading this book, the reader agrees that the author and publisher are not responsible for any losses, injuries, or issues that may result from the application of the information herein, including but not limited to errors, omissions, or inaccuracies.

TABLE OF CONTENTS

TABLE OF CONTENTS

INTRODUCTION

"Every day is a chance to begin again. Don't focus on the failures of yesterday, start today with positive thoughts and expectations."

Catherine Pulsifer

Chair yoga is a type of yoga that is practiced either by sitting on a chair or using a chair for support in standing positions. The traditional yoga poses are simply adapted so they can be practiced with the use of a chair. Chair yoga can be practiced almost anywhere and can easily be adapted for different fitness levels. It's great for individuals who have a limited range of motion, or challenges with balance or strength. For this reason, chair yoga is a suitable and safe practice for seniors.

Chair yoga can improve balance, muscle strength, flexibility, breathing patterns, and mindfulness. It can also reduce stress and support cardiovascular health. Chair yoga has the potential to improve a lot of aspects of your health and well-being, all while being safe and easy to learn.

INTRODUCTION TO THE 28-DAY CHALLENGE

These sequences in this guide will focus on **strength, flexibility, cardiovascular health,** and **balance**. There are also sequences for warming up and cooling down. Each yoga pose has clear instructions and illustrations to help you perform them safely. Modifications are also provided to increase or decrease the challenge according to your needs.

You will also find a 28-day challenge with a daily schedule of exercises to guide you in safe and effective ways of building them into your daily routine. At the end of the 28-day plan, you should begin to see improvements in your fitness and well-being, including an increase in balance, strength, flexibility, and endurance, as well as psychological improvements, including improved tolerance to stress and, in general, a better mood.

Each day's practice will build on the previous one, and become progressively more challenging over time. This will help you to gradually and safely improve as you progress.

IMPORTANCE OF MINDFULNESS, HEALTH, AND WELLNESS

When it comes to yoga, the first thing we tend to think about are physical poses. However, yoga has so much more to offer. First and foremost, mindfulness is a central component of yoga. **Mindfulness is the practice of focusing on the present** without any judgment. For chair yoga, this means try your best to keep your attention on your body when practicing the poses, and come back to your breath when you notice that you start to lose focus.

Another important aspect to mention is that chair yoga should fit into an overall healthy lifestyle. Chair yoga will contribute to improving your physical and mental health, but diet also plays a significant role. Later, we discuss how a balanced diet and a daily walking habit can support your weight loss goals.

Lastly, if you combine breath and relaxation techniques with your chair yoga practice, it will increase your sense of well-being. Chair yoga is an effective part of a holistic approach to a healthy lifestyle. In the next chapter, we will talk about how you can best prepare to begin.

PREPARATION FOR PRACTICE

*"One important key to success is self-confidence.
An important key to self-confidence is preparation."*

Arthur Ashe

It does not require much to begin practicing chair yoga, however, there are still a few things to consider when it comes to space and equipment.

When you set up you practice space, consider:

1. **Find an uncluttered space**. Pick a space with an uncluttered wall where you can prop a chair up against it. Make sure you have enough space to walk around the chair or stretch your legs when seated on the chair.

2. **Exercise on a hard, non-slip surface**. You can put a yoga mat under the chair for non-slip protection. The mat will also come in handy for some of the standing poses as well.

3. **Make the ambiance pleasant**. Pick a space to workout where you will be undisturbed, if possible. Consider using soft lighting, music, candles, crystals, plants, or an essential oil diffuser, if they help you relax and focus.

4. **Adjust the room temperature for comfort**. You don't want to be too cold or too warm during practice.

Next, make sure you have the appropriate equipment for a successful chair yoga practice. You will need:

1. **Use a sturdy, straightback, armless chair**. When seated in the chair, your feet should be able to firmly touch the floor, and you shouldn't feel like your circulation is being cut off at the back of your knees.

2. **Consider props such as yoga blocks or a cushion**. Blocks are optional but can be useful in some poses that require more flexibility. If you don't have yoga blocks, you can also use books as a substitute. A cushion can increase comfort in certain seated poses. Some individuals might prefer a cushion between the backrest and their back during some seated positions.

3. **Add in a yoga mat and blanket**. You don't need a mat for chair yoga, but some people might find it brings more stability under the chair and increases comfort for your feet in standing poses. It is common to cover up with a blanket during the relaxation practice called Savasana pose, so if you have a blanket available, you might choose to use it then.

HEALTH AND SAFETY GUIDELINES

The yoga sequences presented in this book are designed to be safely practiced at home. However, you should always make sure you have clearance from your doctor before undertaking a new exercise program, especially if you have a known medical condition.

To ensure a safe chair yoga practice:

- **Listen to your body.** If a certain pose doesn't feel right or is causing you pain, don't try to force it. Try one of the suggested modifications instead. If that still doesn't work, please move on to another pose.

- **Keep a phone nearby in case of an emergency.** If you live with others, let them know what you will be doing in case you need assistance during your session.

- **Practice yoga barefoot.** If you are not comfortable practicing barefoot, you can wear non-slip athletic shoes. Avoid practicing yoga in socks to avoid slipping.

- **Breathe steadily.** This is especially important in individuals with a known cardiovascular condition or high blood pressure.

Certain positions might not be appropriate for specific health conditions. This is ideally something you can discuss with your healthcare provider. However, here are some of the most common poses to avoid with certain health conditions:

1. Avoid extreme flexion and extension of the spine (rounding your back or arching your back) if you have acute back pain, osteoporosis, or have recently had back surgery.

2. Avoid extreme rotations (deep twists) if you have recently had abdominal surgery, back surgery, injury to your ribs, or suffer from osteoporosis.

3. Avoid side bends if you have recently had back surgery, or an injury to your ribs.

4. Avoid poses that bring the head below the heart if you have high blood pressure, glaucoma, dizziness or vertigo.

It's always best to ask your healthcare provider if you can safely begin a chair yoga practice. Also, listen to your body and adjust according to what feels best for you on a day-to-day basis.

BE SAFE AND EFFECTIVE

To ensure your safety and effectiveness while performing these strength sequences, follow the tips below.

1. **Respect your limits**
   When it comes to building strength, more is not always better. If there is a specific pose that is difficult to perform, or if you need a break, listen to your body. You will be able to build strength much more efficiently from a place of comfort and control. If you control the movement you are doing, it will be easier to activate the right muscles and avoid strain that might cause injury.

2. **Stay consistent**
   You can't expect to build strength if you rarely perform strengthening routines. Aim to include a strength sequence two times per week. By doing so, you will be able to increase the challenge over time and build up your muscle tissue.

3. **Allow time for recovery**
   Although we encourage consistency, we also don't want to overdo it. It's possible that after a strength routine, you feel sore in comparison to doing a routine that focuses more on flexibility or cardio. It's important to allow time for recovery before your next workout. You want to leave at least one day of rest in between each strength-building session. You can either take a rest day, or do another yoga sequence that targets another fitness component such as flexibility or cardio.

4. **Be mindful of your alignment**
   Finally, proper alignment matters when trying to build muscle strength. Each pose targets a specific set of muscles. For example, when a pose requires the hip to be turned out it will activate the glutes. It's important to pay attention and carefully adjust each pose as instructed to get the most out of the pose and build up the right muscles.

SET YOUR GOALS AND INTENTIONS

Although they can seem interchangeable, a *goal* and an *intention* are different concepts, especially when it comes to yoga. A *goal* is typically something specific and measurable that you wish to accomplish in the future. An *intention* reflects how you want to be present during your practice. Intentions compliment a mindfulness practice, because they help to remind you of the mindset that you would like to cultivate in your daily life, and they remind you to pay attention to the quality of your thoughts and feelings as you practice.

We encourage you to set a long-term goal for your 28-day challenge, and set intentions for each day that you practice yoga during the 28-day challenge. To set a goal for your 28-day chair yoga challenge, we suggest using the SMART criteria which is a popular framework used across many disciplines for effective goal setting (Doran, 1981).

The SMART acronym stands for:

S=Specific   **M**=Measurable **A**=Achievable **R**=Relevant   **T**=Time-bound

Here is an example of what a SMART goal could look like in the context of a 28-day chair yoga challenge:

"I will improve my ability to perform daily activities like lifting my knees higher, bending more easily, and requiring less support. I will do this by completing the 28-day chair yoga challenge."

This goal is specific, time-bound, and relevant: it will help you be more functional in your everyday life and increase your independence.

Specific: You will improve your ability to lift your knees, bend, and balance.

Measurable: You can observe how much easier it is to move in these precise ways.

Achievable: You can follow the 28-day plan and assess your improvement at the end.

Relevant: Your goal aligns with a valuable plan to improve function and independence in daily activities.

Time-Bound: You set a specific time frame of 28 days to accomplish the goal.

Your SMART goal will most likely be different from this one, but you can still use the SMART structure to make it focused and achievable. As you set your SMART goal, be honest with yourself and consider your current physical condition. Also, consider what aspect of your health, whether physical, mental, or both, is a priority for you right now. Make your goal something you can genuinely commit to working toward.

To set an intention, the process will be slightly different. Typically, intentions are set at the beginning of practice when you ground yourself and take a few deep breaths. Once your intention is set, try to remind yourself of it throughout your session, especially when you find yourself losing focus.

Here are a few ideas on ways to set an intention:

- Think about what your body or mind needs on a given day. For example, your intention could be compassion, gratitude, or self-love.

- Choose an affirmation for your intention. For example, "I choose peace," or "I am resilient."

- Dedicate your practice to someone. For example, your intention could be to generate courage for someone who is going through a difficult time, or, to send love to someone who means a lot to you.

You now have all the tools you need to begin learning the chair yoga exercises described in the next chapters.

WARMING UP AND BREATHING

"Breathe. Let go. And remind yourself that this very moment is the only one you know you have for sure."

Oprah Winfrey

THE IMPORTANCE OF WARM-UPS

Warming up at the beginning of an exercise session can create many positive physiological changes in our bodies. Warm-ups enhance blood flow, which delivers more oxygen to the muscles, improves nerve function, and reduces the risk of injury. Warm-ups also help you focus during the activity, which can have positive psychological benefits including increased mindfulness and a greater sense of enjoyment (McGowan et al., 2015 and Woods et al., 2007).

You want to prepare the body physically and mentally for your practice. It's important to **keep the intensity low and avoid exhausting yourself** right from the beginning. Take a few minutes to warm up with slow, gentle poses before moving into the more challenging portion of your workout.

THE ROLE OF BREATHING IN YOGA

Pranayama is the Sanskrit term for breath control. More specifically, *prana* means *vital energy,* and *yama* means *control*. Pranayama is an integral part of any yoga practice, because breathing plays a very important role in moderating your energy throughout the session. **Yoga links the breath to each movement,** and specific breathing techniques can be used to energize the body or calm the nervous system down, as needed.

Breathing is also used as part of meditation. Research has also found evidence of multiple health benefits of yogic breathing for patients with specific health conditions. A systematic review by Jayawardena et al., published in the *International Journal of Yoga* (2020) found that yogic breathing techniques were linked to less frequent and less severe asthma attacks for patients with bronchial asthma, and less fatigue and anxiety in patients with cancer and cardiovascular disease.

The yoga sequences included in this book include cues on when to inhale and exhale to help you become aware of how you breathe as you move from pose to pose. In general, the rule is simple: try to **inhale as you expand and open up in a pose, and exhale when you contract and bend.** We will also touch on breath awareness as part of the cool down and meditation sequences.

BASIC CHAIR YOGA WARM-UP SERIES

Perform the following warm-up series at the beginning of your yoga practice to prepare your body. These sequences are designed to flow, so you do not need to hold the positions for a long time; try to keep moving gently and mindfully from one pose to the next, while concentrating on breathing steadily as you move. The Sun Salutation, which appears in the next chapter, also makes an excellent warm-up exercise.

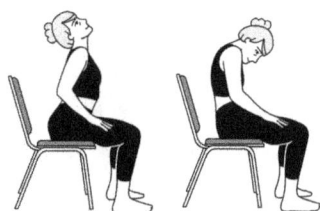

SEATED CAT
AND COW POSE

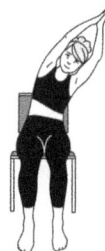

SEATED SIDE
BEND POSE

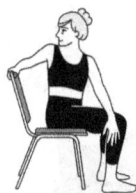

CHAIR SEATED
TWIST

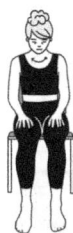

SEATED
NECK ROLLS

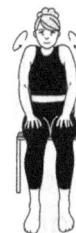

SEATED
SHOULDER ROLLS

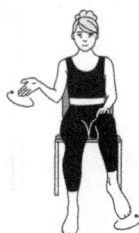

SEATED ANKLE
AND WRIST ROTATIONS

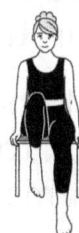

SEATED
MARCHES

Seated Cat and Cow Pose

- Sit tall in a chair, place your feet hip-distance apart, and rest your hands on your thighs.

- Inhale as you arch your back and lift your sternum toward the ceiling for Cow Pose.

- Exhale as you round your back and bring your chin toward your chest for Cat Pose.

- Move back and forth between Cat and Cow Pose while syncing your movement to your breath. Repeat for 10 repetitions.

- Inhale and return to a neutral seated position.

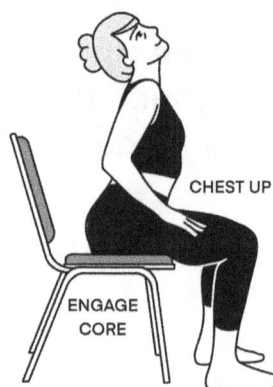

CHEST UP

ENGAGE CORE

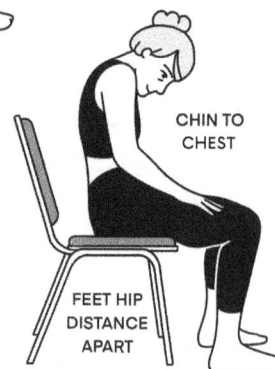

CHIN TO CHEST

FEET HIP DISTANCE APART

Seated Side Bend Pose

- Inhale, lengthen through your spine, and lift your arms overhead.

- Interlace your fingers while pointing your thumb and index fingers.

- Exhale and stretch to the right.

- Both feet should be actively pressing into the ground.

- Exhale into a side bend and then inhale and rise back to the center and release your arms down to your sides.

- Repeat five times on each side.

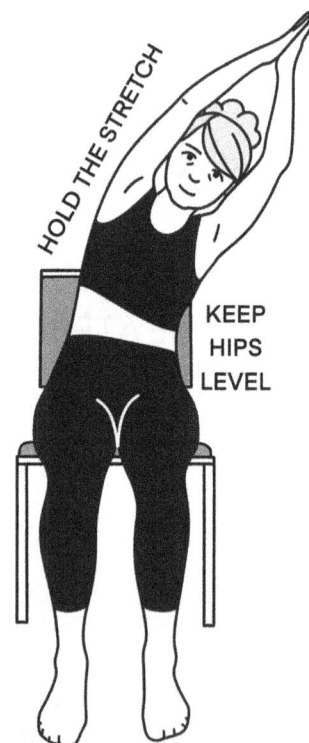

HOLD THE STRETCH

KEEP HIPS LEVEL

Chair Seated Twist

- Exhale and twist to the right side.

- Hold onto the back of the chair with your right hand, and press your left hand into your right thigh.

- Inhale, lengthen your spine, engage your core and exhale to twist a little further.

- Lift your chest, relax your shoulders, and deepen the twist.

- Alternate between twisting on an exhale and coming back to center on an inhale.

- Repeat five times on each side.

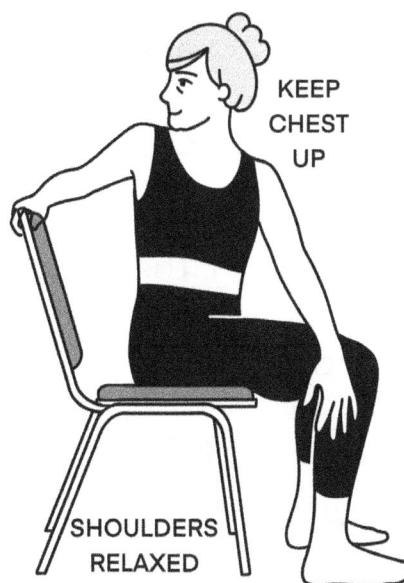

KEEP CHEST UP

SHOULDERS RELAXED

SUGGESTED MODIFICATIONS

To **decrease the challenge**, do not twist as far.

Seated Neck Rolls

- Breathe steadily and bring your chin toward your chest.

- Slowly roll your head forward from left to right in a half circle.

- Repeat five times in each direction.

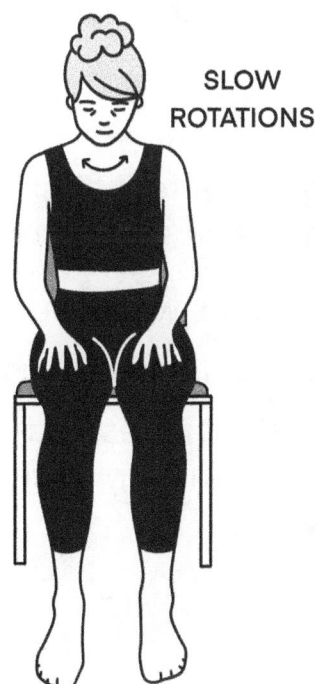

SLOW ROTATIONS

Seated Shoulder Rolls

- Breathe steadily and roll your shoulders up, back, and down in a circular motion.

- Repeat 5-10 times in one direction, then reverse the direction for another 5-10 repetitions.

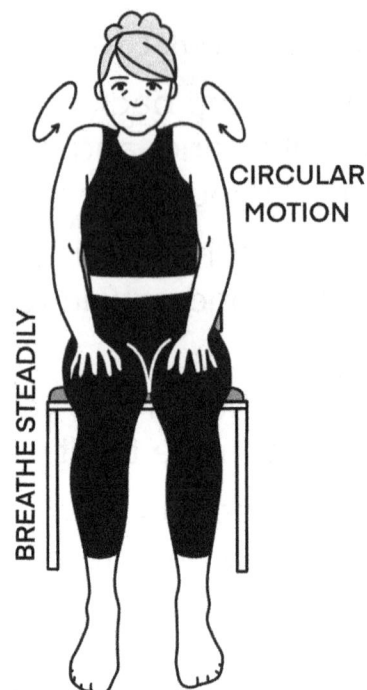

CIRCULAR MOTION

BREATHE STEADILY

Seated Ankle and Wrist Rotations

- Breathe steadily, lift your right foot off the floor, and make a few circles with your ankle in each direction.

- Repeat with your left ankle.

- Then, lift both hands and make circles with your wrists five times in each direction.

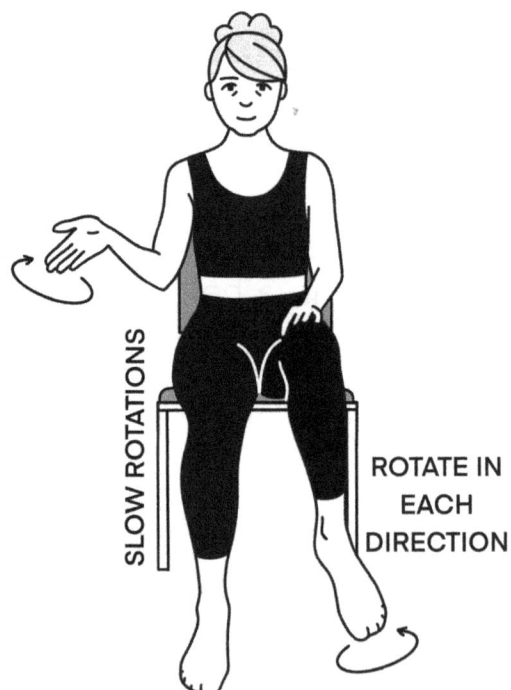

SLOW ROTATIONS

ROTATE IN EACH DIRECTION

Seated Marches

- Bring both hands to the seat on either side of your thighs, then inhale to lengthen your spine.

- Exhale to lift your right knee toward your chest, then inhale to lower your leg back down.

- Repeat with alternating legs for 10 repetitions on each side.

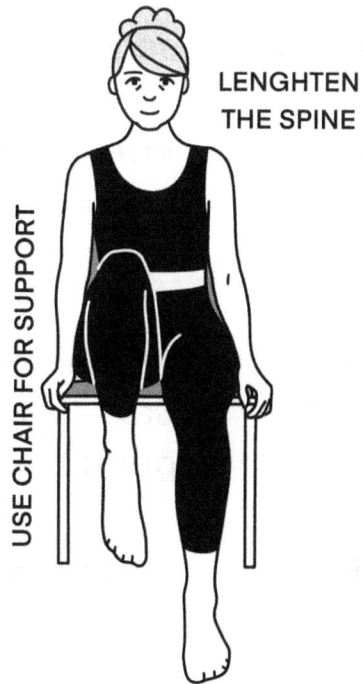

LENGHTEN THE SPINE

USE CHAIR FOR SUPPORT

CONCLUSION

In the next chapter, we will discuss the benefits of the Sun and Moon Salutations, as well as how you can integrate them into your yoga practice.

BONUS CONTENT

We want to see you achieve your goals. To help, I've included bonus resources with you in mind: Easy-to-follow Video Tutorials, Printable Trackers, Illustrated Posters and more.

BONUS #1 | **Video Tutorials** - Get unlimited access to easy-to-follow video tutorials that guide you through how to do every exercise in the book.

BONUS #2 | **Printable Trackers and Illustrated Posters** - Stay motivated and track your progress with weekly printable guides.

BONUS #3 | **7-Step Guide to Kicking Fear and Anxiety** - This guide helps you build your confidence and commit to establishing a new wellness routine.

BONUS #4 | **Guided Meditations** - Immerse yourself in calming guided meditations designed to support your wellness journey.

BONUS #5 | **Facebook Community** - Connect with like-minded individuals, share your progress, ask questions, and receive ongoing support and motivation from both peers and experts.

The LINK and PIN code to unlock your bonus is on the last page of this book.

These bonuses are **FREE** and designed to **help you achieve your goals**.

EXPLORING THE SUN AND MOON SALUTATIONS

4

"Don't compare your life to others. There's no comparison between the sun and the moon, they shine when it's their time."

Unknown

In this chapter, you will learn the Sun and Moon Salutations, which are sequences that encourage you to find your center, be present in the moment, and link your breath to your movement. Typically, Sun Salutations feel more energizing, and Moon Salutations feel more calming.

The Sun and Moon Salutations are both powerful sequences that allow you time to look inward, be present, and practice poses that increase feelings of energy, harmony, and balance.

SUN SALUTATION SERIES: A GENTLE START

Sun Salutations are known as *Surya Namaskar* in Sanskrit. *Surya* means *sun* and *Namaskar* means *I pay my salutations*. Therefore, *Surya Namaskar* (Sun Salutation) means "to bow to the sun, or to show gratitude to the sun."

In most cultures, the sun is a symbol of energy and life. You will notice that the sun salutation energizes and heats in the body. For this reason, this sequence is typically done a few times at the beginning of a yoga practice as part of the warm-up, but it can just as well be a stand-alone practice.

The Sun Salutation improves strength and flexibility, energizes your mind and body, provides the time to cultivate awareness and gratitude, and harmonizes your mind and body by linking your breath to movement. Three variations of the Sun Salutation (A, B, and C) exist. For this book, we will focus on a seated variation of Sun Salutation A, a sequence of poses that align with the breath and flow gently. We will also provide modifications for some of the poses that might be challenging, so that you can practice whichever variation feels best for you.

SEATED SUN SALUTATION SERIES

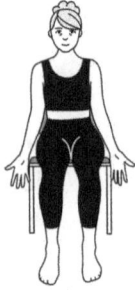

**SEATED
MOUNTAIN POSE**

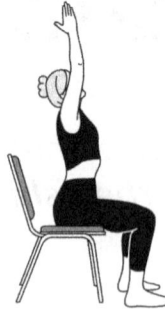

**SEATED UPWARD
HANDS POSE**

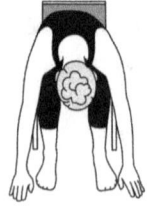

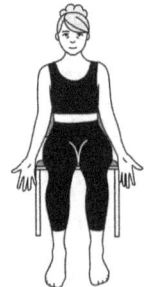

**SEATED
FORWARD FOLD**

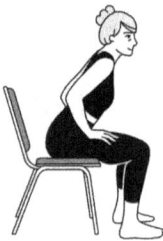

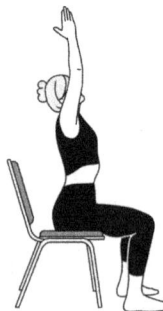

**SEATED
HALFWAY LIFT**

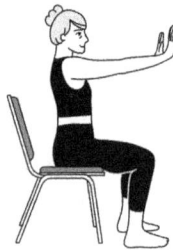

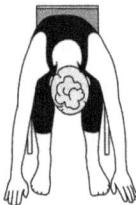

**SEATED
PLANK POSE**

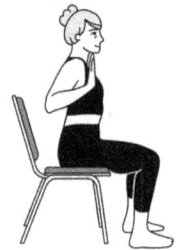

**SEATED FOUR-
LIMBED STAFF POSE**

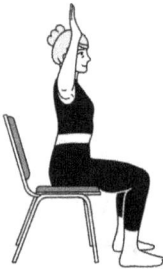

**SEATED UPWARD-
FACING DOG**

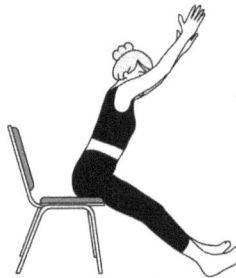

**SEATED DOWNWARD-
FACING DOG**

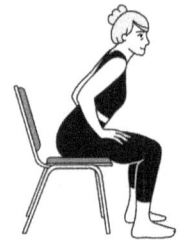

**SEATED
HALFWAY LIFT**

**SEATED
FORWARD FOLD**

**SEATED UPWARD
HANDS POSE**

**SEATED
MOUNTAIN POSE**

Seated Mountain Pose

- Begin seated with your back straight.

- Place your feet hip-distance apart, and press the soles of your feet into the ground. (Feel "all four corners" of your feet pressing firmly down).

- Your arms should be relaxed by your side with palms facing forward.

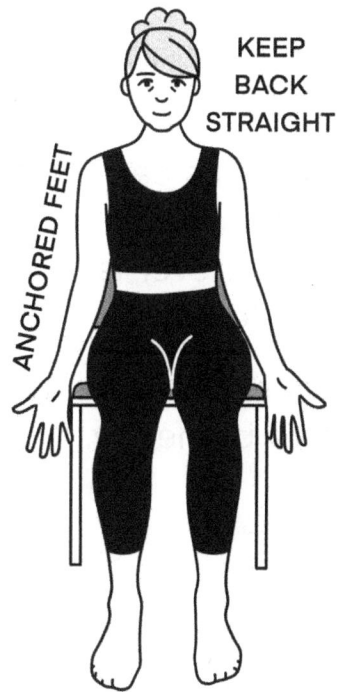

KEEP BACK STRAIGHT

ANCHORED FEET

Seated Upward Hands Pose

- Inhale and lift your arms overhead while gazing towards your hands, and touch your palms together.

- Lengthen your spine, and gently arch your back at the end of the movement.

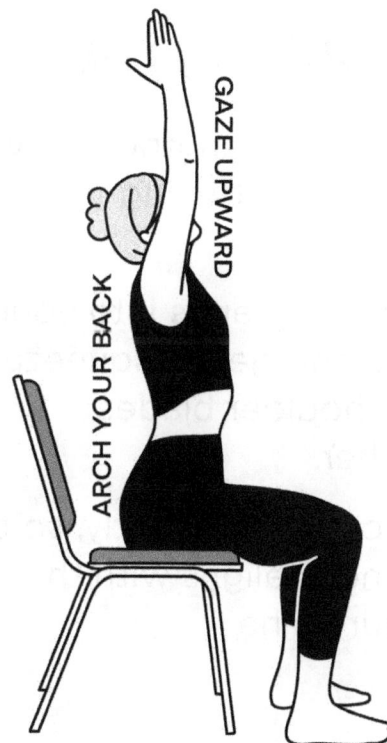

GAZE UPWARD

ARCH YOUR BACK

Seated Forward Fold

- Lengthen your spine and exhale forward.

- Your fingertips can touch the ground, or rest on your thighs, whichever is more comfortable.

- Relax your shoulders, and let your head be heavy.

SHOULDERS RELAXED

LENGTHEN YOUR SPINE

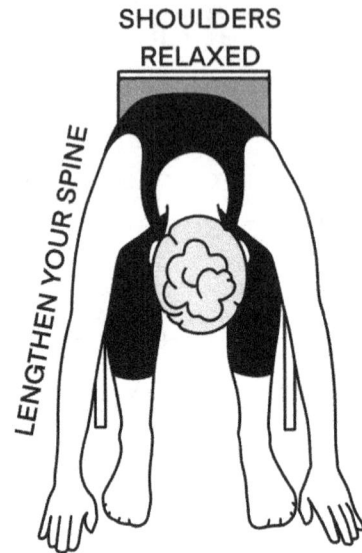

Seated Halfway Lift

- Inhale while lengthening your spine and flattening your back.

- Press your hands into your thighs and gently squeeze your shoulder blades together.

- Lift your head slightly, so that your neck aligns with the rest of your spine.

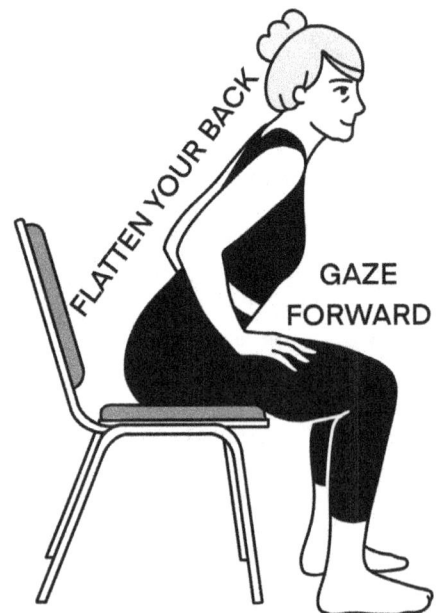

FLATTEN YOUR BACK

GAZE FORWARD

Seated Plank Pose

- Exhale and lengthen your spine so that you are in a tall, seated position.

- Bring your arms straight out in front of you with your wrists aligned at shoulder height.

- Imagine you are pressing your palms into a wall in front of you.

- Pull your navel in toward your spine to engage your core.

- Keep your neck in line with the rest of your spine as you hold the position.

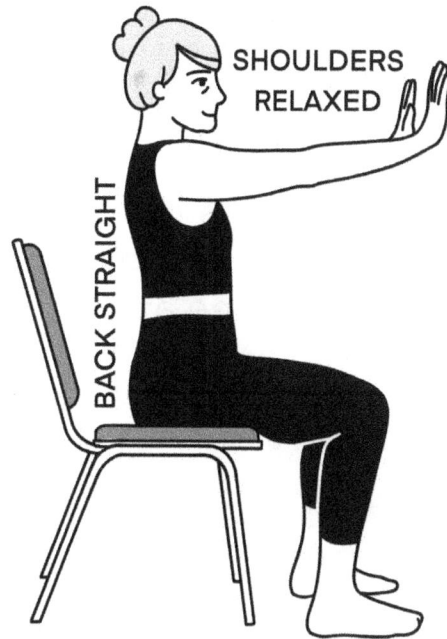

Seated Four-Limbed Staff Pose

- Exhale as you bend your elbows and bring your hands next to your rib cage at shoulder height.

- Your body should form a straight line.

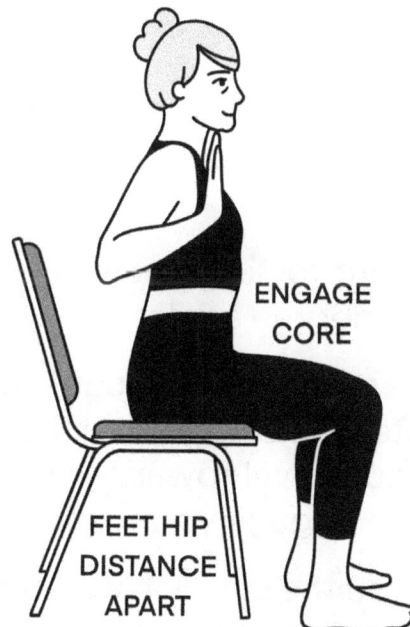

Seated Upward-Facing Dog

- Inhale, open your chest, and arch your back.

- Extend your arms out to the side, with your elbows bent at 90 degree angle.

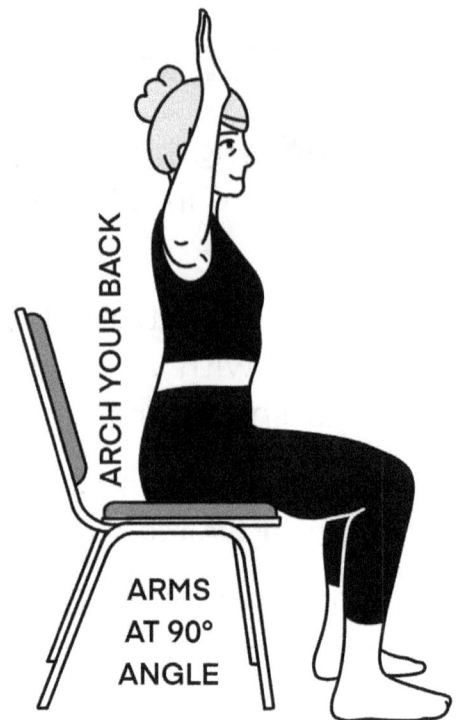

ARCH YOUR BACK

ARMS
AT 90°
ANGLE

Seated Downward-Facing Dog

- Exhale and extend your arms, keeping your arms in line with your ears, palms facing in front of you.

- Straighten your legs in front of you, and rest your heels on the ground.

- Lean your torso forward at a 45 degree angle.

- Keep a slight bend in your knees to protect your lower back, and pull your navel toward your spine to engage your core.

- Keep your head in line with the rest of your spine and hold the pose for a few breaths.

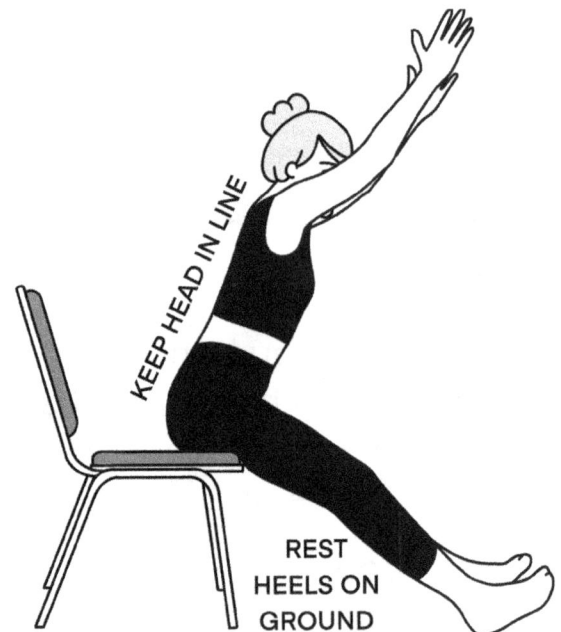

KEEP HEAD IN LINE

REST
HEELS ON
GROUND

SUGGESTED MODIFICATIONS

To **decrease the challenge**, bend your knees, or modify how high you lift your arms.

Seated Halfway Lift

- Inhale as you bring your hands to your thighs.

- Bend your knees and press your feet into the mat.

- Gently squeeze your shoulder blades together.

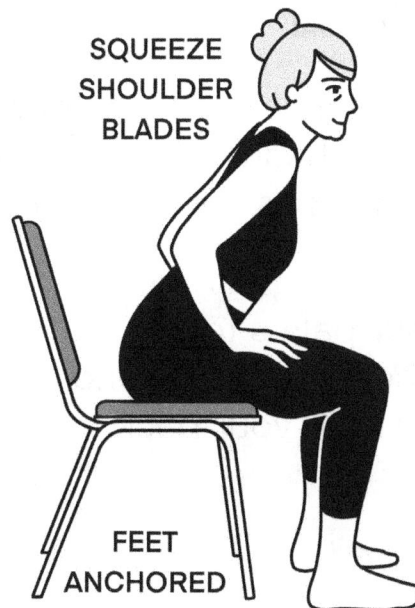

SQUEEZE SHOULDER BLADES

FEET ANCHORED

Seated Forward Fold

- Exhale while folding forward; lengthen your spine.

- Rest your fingertips on the ground, or on your thighs, whichever is more comfortable.

- Relax your shoulders, and let your head be heavy.

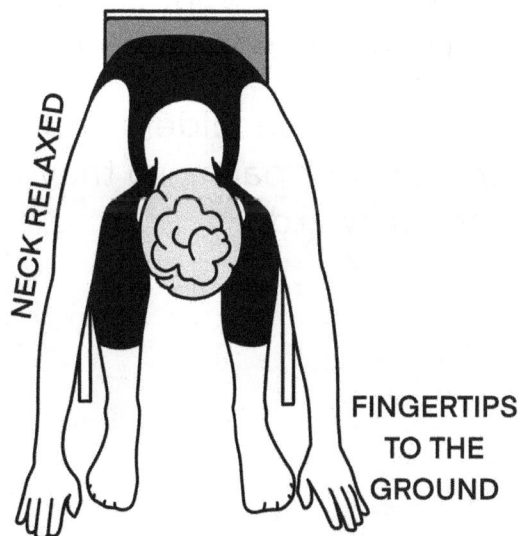

NECK RELAXED

FINGERTIPS TO THE GROUND

Seated Upward Hands Pose

- Inhale while extending your arms overhead; gaze toward your hands as you lift your arms.

- As your palms touch, lengthen your spine and gently arch your back.

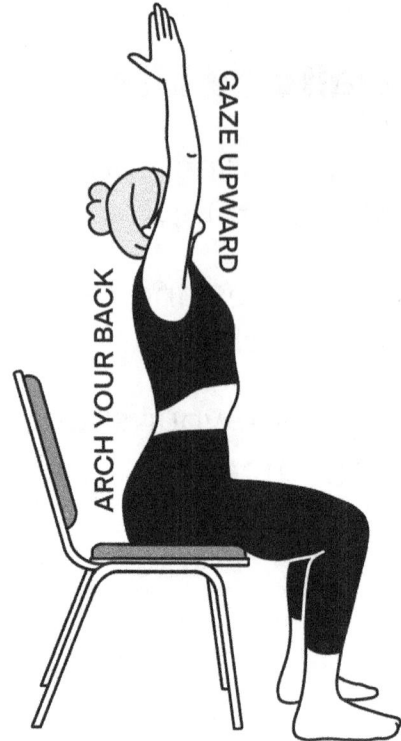

GAZE UPWARD

ARCH YOUR BACK

Seated Mountain Pose

- Exhale as you release your arms down to your side and finish the Sun Salutation.

- Relax your shoulders and rotate your palms so they face forward.

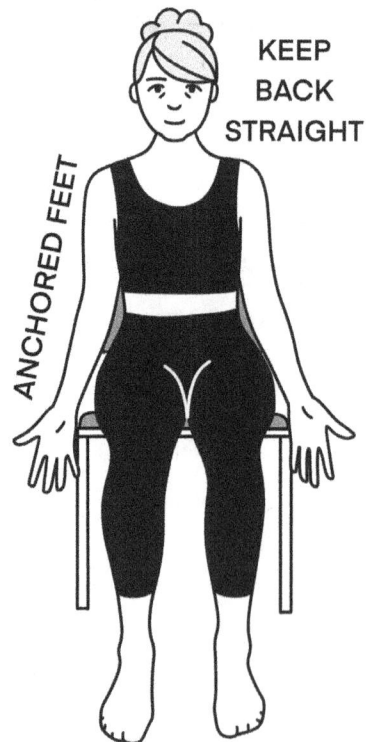

KEEP BACK STRAIGHT

ANCHORED FEET

SEATED MOON SALUTATION SERIES: FOR MIND-BODY HARMONY

Moon Salutations are known as *Chandra Namaskar* in Sanskrit. *Chandra* means *bright* or *shining*. *Namaskar* means *I pay my salutations*. In other words, *Chandra Namaskar* (Moon Salutation) means "to bow to the moon or honor the moon."

As we know, the moon goes through different cycles. The Moon Salutation reminds us that life, like the moon, also moves in different phases. The Moon Salutation is made up of poses that resemble different phases of the moon cycle, and it is meant to be calming and restorative. Therefore, it is often practiced before sleep or as part of a cool-down. It can also be done as a stand-alone practice any time during the day to create mind-body harmony, and relax or calm the nervous system.

The Moon Salutation improves flexibility, creates a sense of relaxation, and provides time to restore and reflect.

Many variations of the Moon Salutation exist; in this book, we present a seated chair version of the Moon Salutation series. We also provide modifications for some of the poses that might be challenging, so that you can practice whichever variation feels best.

The directions below include cues for performing the sequence on one side of the body, and then the other. Be sure to stretch both sides of the body equally for a balanced practice.

SEATED MOON SALUTATION SERIES

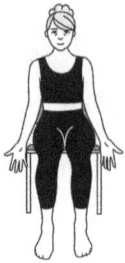

SEATED
MOUNTAIN POSE

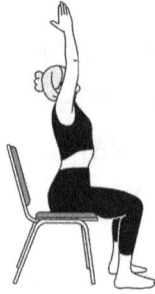

SEATED UPWARD
HANDS POSE

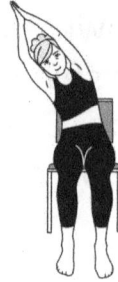

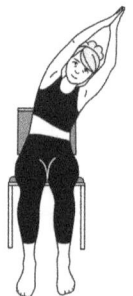

SEATED SIDE
BEND POSE

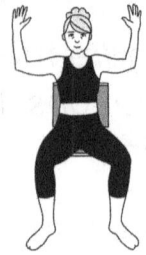

SEATED
GODDESS POSE

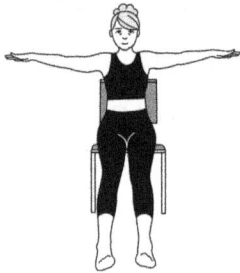

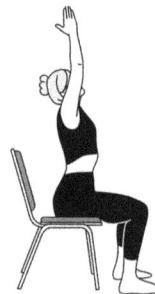

SEATED
FIVE-POINTED
STAR POSE

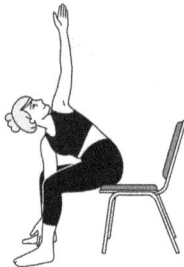

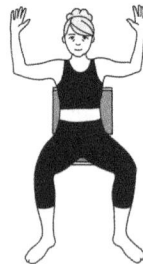

SEATED
TRIANGLE POSE

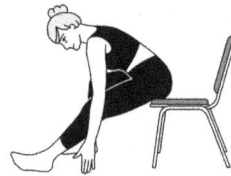

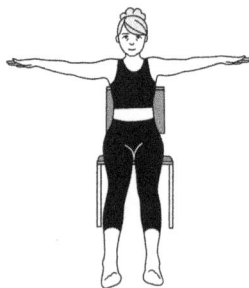

SEATED
PYRAMID POSE

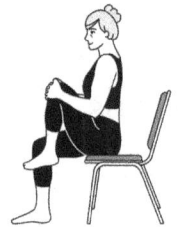

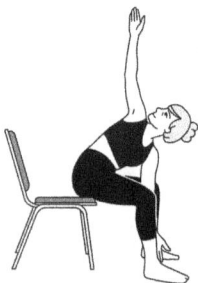

SEATED
LOW LUNGE

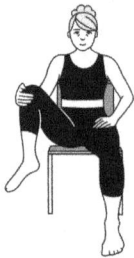

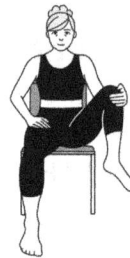

SEATED
SIDE LUNGE

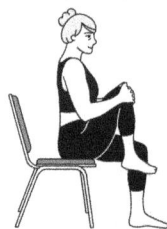

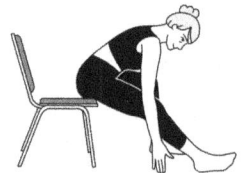

SEATED
LOW LUNGE

SEATED
SIDE LUNGE

SEATED
PYRAMID POSE

SEATED
TRIANGLE
POSE

SEATED
FIVE-POINTED
STAR POSE

SEATED
GODDESS
POSE

SEATED
UPWARD
HANDS POSE

SEATED
SIDE BEND
POSE

Seated Mountain Pose

- Begin seated on your chair with your back straight.

- Place your feet hip-distance apart, and press the soles of your feet into the ground. (Feel "all four corners" of your feet pressing firmly down).

- Your arms should be relaxed by your side with palms facing forward.

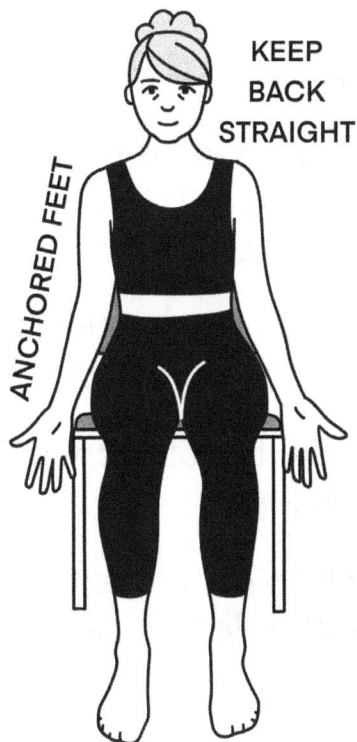

KEEP BACK STRAIGHT

ANCHORED FEET

Seated Upward Hands Pose

- Inhale, lift your arms overhead while gazing toward your hands, and touch your palms together.

- Lengthen your spine, and gently arch your back.

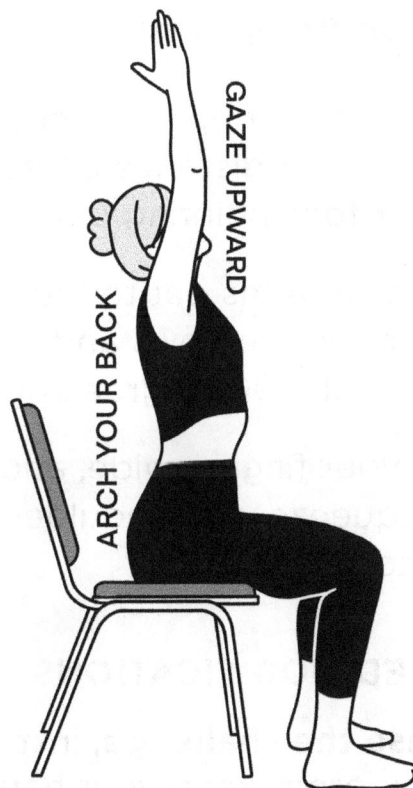

GAZE UPWARD

ARCH YOUR BACK

Seated Side Bend Pose

- Begin with your arms lifted over in Seated Upward Hands Pose. Exhale and extend to the left.

- Both feet should be actively pressing into the ground.

- Hold and feel the stretch in the right side body.

- Inhale back to center, extend to the left, then release your arms.

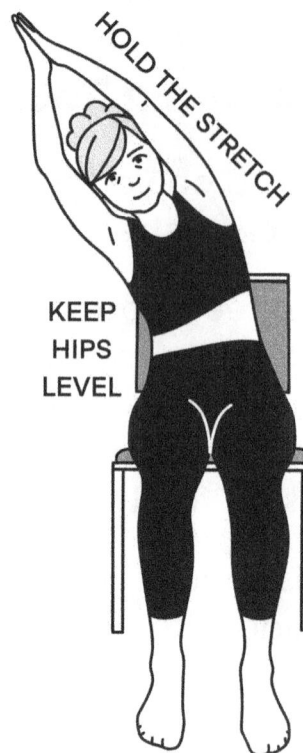

HOLD THE STRETCH

KEEP HIPS LEVEL

Seated Goddess Pose

- Exhale as you bring your feet wider than hip-distance apart with your toes pointing out.

- Extend your arms out to the sides with your elbows and shoulders at a 90-degree angle.

- Spread your fingers wide, and gently squeeze your shoulder blades together.

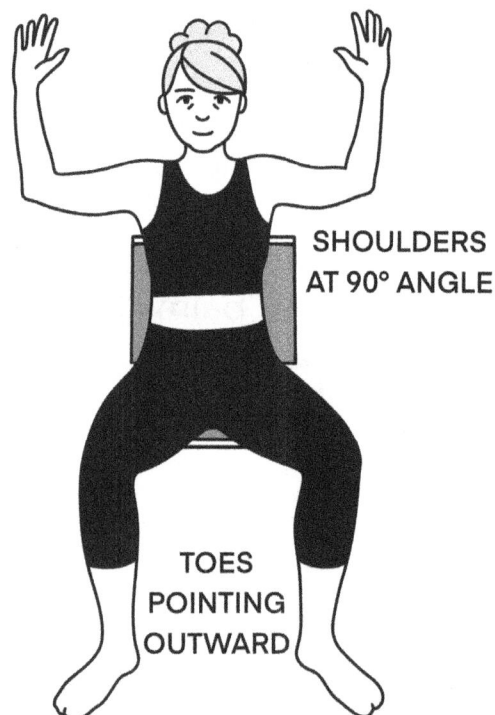

SUGGESTED MODIFICATIONS

To **decrease the challenge**, instead of raising your arms, keep your hands together at your heart center. To **increase the challenge**, push through the soles of your feet and raise your buttocks off of the chair.

SHOULDERS AT 90° ANGLE

TOES POINTING OUTWARD

Seated Five-Pointed Star Pose

- Inhale as you straighten your legs and rest your heels on the ground.

- Keep a slight bend in your knees to protect your low back.

- Extend your arms out to the side at shoulder height, and relax your shoulders.

- Lengthen through your spine and gaze forward.

- Hold the pose, and breathe.

DON'T LOCK YOUR KNEES

SHOULDERS RELAXED

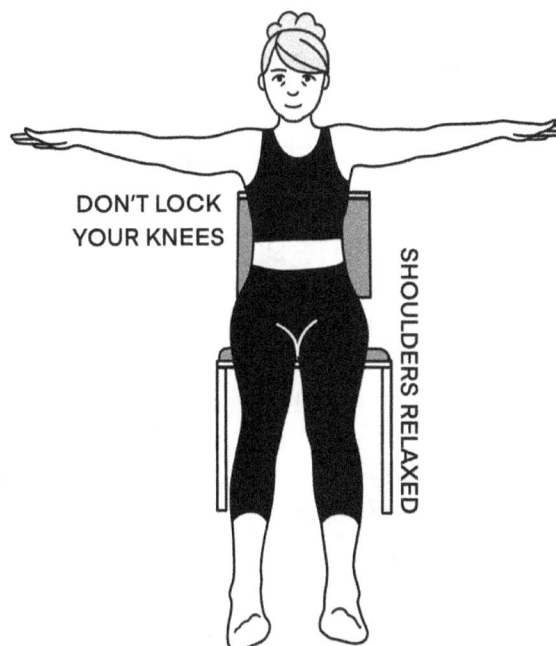

Seated Triangle Pose

- Exhale as you rotate your torso to the right while keeping your arms outstretched.

- Slowly bend down to bring the fingertips of your left hand toward the ground on the inside of your left foot.

- Reach your right arm toward the ceiling.

- Align your neck with the rest of the spine, and look toward your right hand if possible. Otherwise, you can look down or straight ahead, wherever it feels best for your neck.

- Hold the pose and inhale as you stretch both arms in opposite directions.

- Repeat on the other side.

ALIGN NECK WITH SPINE

REACH UPWARD

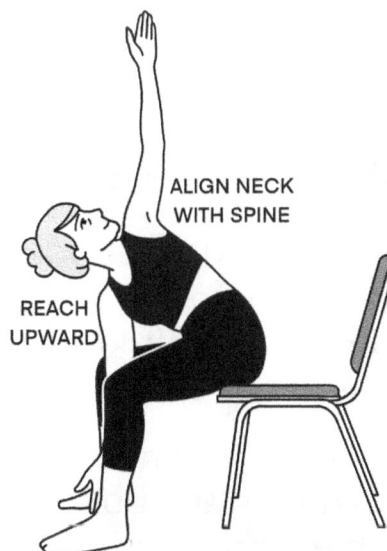

SUGGESTED MODIFICATIONS

To **decrease the challenge**, rest your elbow on your thigh instead of reaching your fingertips towards the ground. You can also rest your hand on a yoga block for extra support.

Seated Pyramid Pose

- Exhale, extend your left leg out in front of you, and press your heel into the ground.

- Hinge at the hips and fold forward while lengthening through your spine.

- Keep your torso parallel to the floor, and rest both hands on the floor, on either side of your left leg.

- Direct your gaze toward the floor.

- Return to the center, and then repeat on the other side.

LENGTHEN THE SPINE

HEEL PRESSED TO THE GROUND

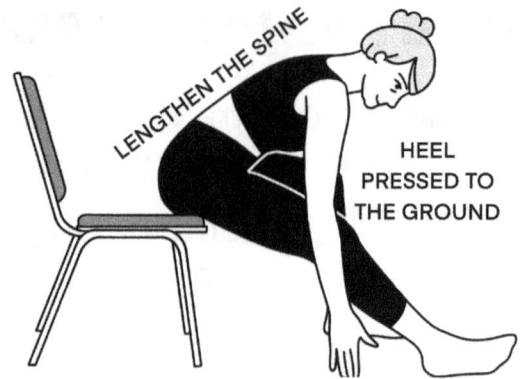

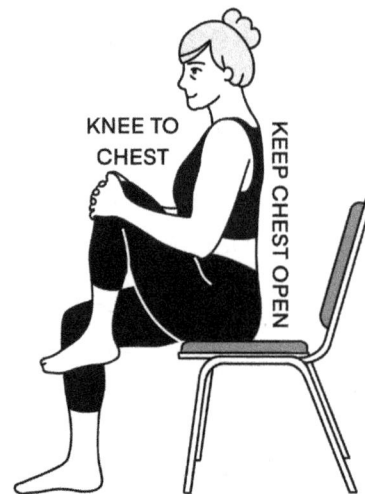

SUGGESTED MODIFICATIONS

To **decrease the challenge**, rest your hands on your shin or thigh instead of on the floor. You can also use a yoga block on either side of your foot to support your hands, if that feels more comfortable.

Seated Low Lunge

- Inhale as you press your right foot into the ground and raise the left knee toward your chest.

- Hold your left knee with both hands and pull your thigh toward your chest.

- Lengthen through your spine and open your chest.

- Gaze forward and hold the pose while you breathe.

- Release your leg, and repeat on the other side.

KNEE TO CHEST

KEEP CHEST OPEN

SUGGESTED MODIFICATIONS

To **decrease the challenge**, modify how closely you pull your thigh towards your chest, and reduce how far you extend it to the side. You can also hold onto the back of your thigh instead of the front of the knee, if that feels more comfortable.

Seated Side Lunge

- Hold onto your left leg, exhale and extend your left leg out to the left side while keeping your right foot anchored to the ground.

- Expand your chest and look forward.

- Inhale and open your chest even more: hold the pose and breathe, then exhale and gently release your left leg and repeat on the other side.

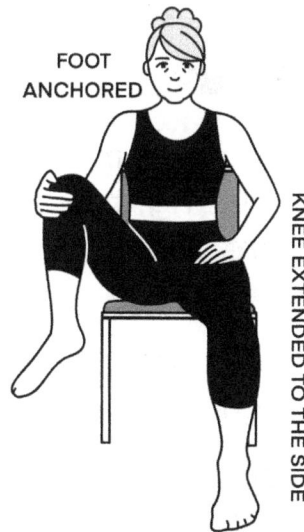

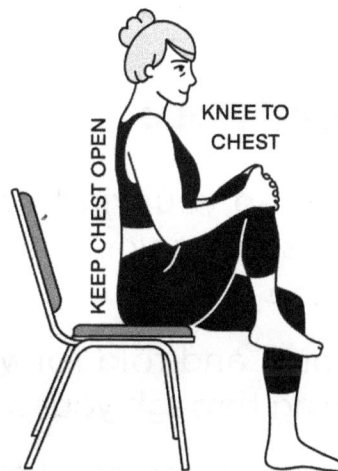

FOOT ANCHORED

KNEE EXTENDED TO THE SIDE

SUGGESTED MODIFICATIONS

To **decrease the challenge**, modify how closely you pull your thigh towards your chest. You can also hold onto the back of your thigh instead of the front of the knee, if that feels more comfortable.

Seated Low Lunge

- Inhale as you press your left foot into the ground and raise the right knee toward your chest.

- Hold your right knee with both hands and pull your thigh toward your chest.

- Lengthen through your spine and open your chest.

- Gaze forward and hold the pose while you breathe.

- Release your leg, and repeat on the other side.

KEEP CHEST OPEN

KNEE TO CHEST

SUGGESTED MODIFICATIONS

To **decrease the challenge**, modify how closely you pull your thigh towards your chest, and reduce how far you extend it to the side. You can also hold onto the back of your thigh instead of the front of the knee, if that feels more comfortable.

Seated Side Lunge

- Exhale as you bring your right leg out to the right side while you are still holding onto it.

- Keep your left foot firmly pressed into the floor.

- Open your chest, lengthen your spine, and maintain a steady forward gaze while you hold the pose.

- Release your right leg, come back to center, and repeat on the other side.

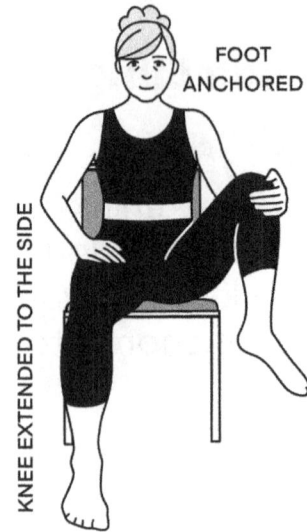

FOOT ANCHORED

KNEE EXTENDED TO THE SIDE

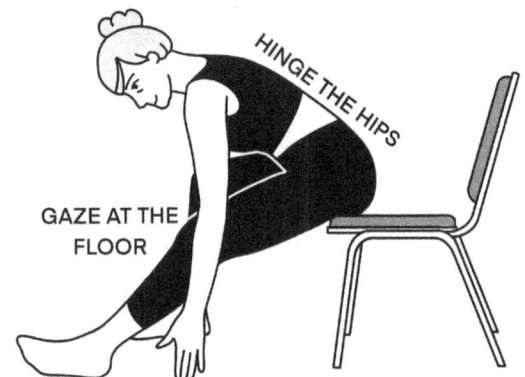

SUGGESTED MODIFICATIONS

To **decrease the challenge**, modify how closely you bring your thigh toward your chest and how far you extend it out to the side. You can also hold onto the back of your thigh instead of the front of the knee, if that feels more comfortable.

Seated Pyramid Pose

- Exhale and extend your right leg in front of you so that your heel rests against the floor.

- Hinge at the hips and fold forward while lengthening through your spine.

- You can keep your torso parallel to the floor, or fold deeper if you prefer.

- Rest both hands on the floor on either side of your right leg, and direct your gaze toward the floor, if it feels comfortable.

- Return to center, and repeat on the other side.

HINGE THE HIPS

GAZE AT THE FLOOR

SUGGESTED MODIFICATIONS

To **decrease the challenge**, place your hands on your shin or on your thigh instead of on the floor. You can also rest your hands on a yoga block on either side of your foot for extra support.

Seated Triangle Pose

- Press both feet into the ground hip-distance apart, and inhale as you rise up.

- Lengthen through your spine and stretch your arms out to the side at shoulder height.

- Keep your arms extended and exhale as you rotate your torso to the left.

- Slowly move into a side bend and bring your right fingertips toward the ground on the inside of your right foot.

- Your left arm should be reaching toward the ceiling.

- Look toward your left hand, if possible. Otherwise, you can look down or straight ahead, whichever feels more comfortable.

- Keep your neck aligned with the rest of your spine, and inhale as you stretch both arms in opposite directions.

- Return to center, and repeat on the other side.

ALIGN NECK WITH SPINE

REACH UPWARD

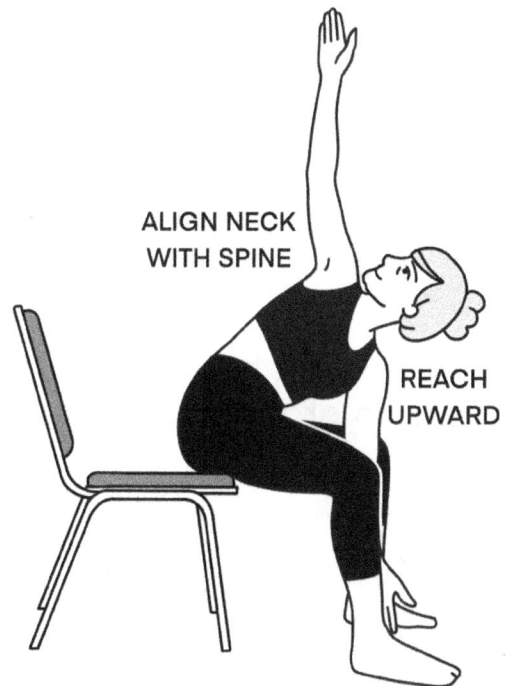

SUGGESTED MODIFICATIONS

To **decrease the challenge**, rest your elbow on your thigh instead of reaching your fingertips towards the ground. You can also rest your hand on a yoga block for extra support.

Seated Five-Pointed Star Pose

- Exhale and lift into a tall seated position.

- Inhale as you straighten your legs and press your heels into the floor.

- Keep a slight bend in your knees to protect your low back.

- Extend your arms out to the side at shoulder height, and relax the shoulders.

- Lengthen through your spine, direct your gaze forward, and breathe as you hold the pose.

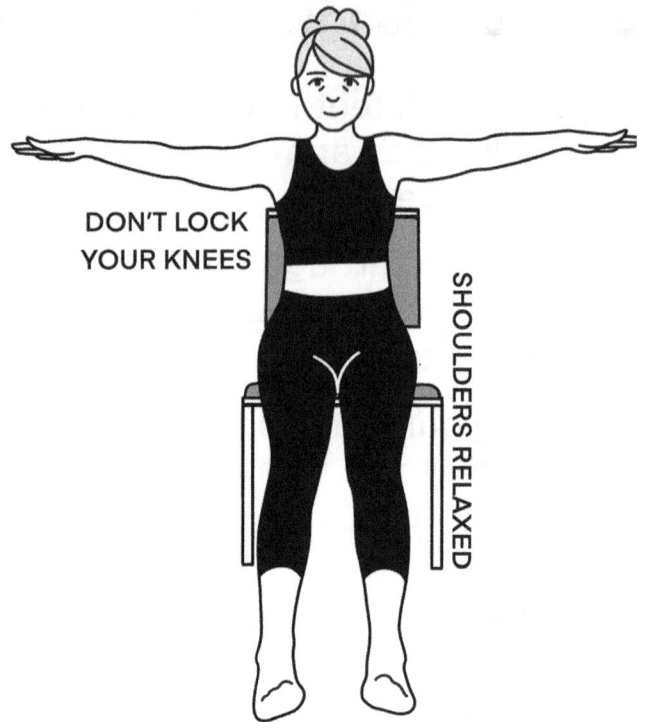

DON'T LOCK YOUR KNEES

SHOULDERS RELAXED

Seated Goddess Pose

- Exhale and place your feet wider than hip-distance apart with your toes pointing out.

- Lift your arms out to the sides so your elbows and shoulders are at a 90-degree angle, like a cactus.

- Spread your fingers wide and gently squeeze your shoulder blades together.

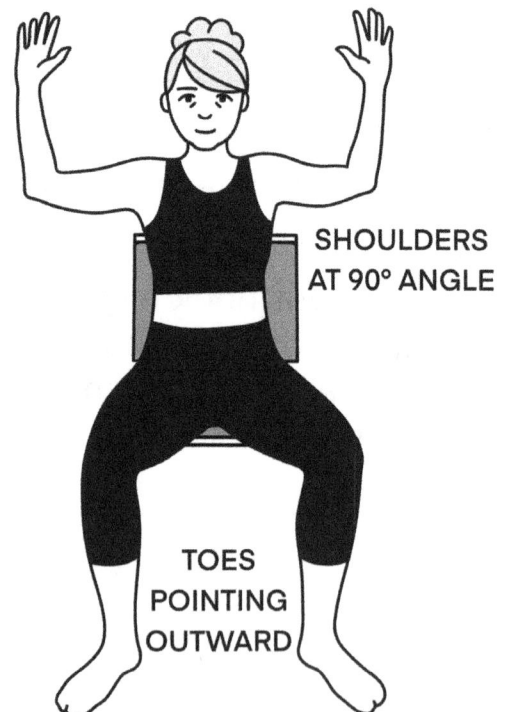

SUGGESTED MODIFICATIONS

To **decrease the challenge**, keep your hands together at the heart center. To **increase the challenge**, push through your feet and try to lift your buttocks from the chair.

SHOULDERS AT 90° ANGLE

TOES POINTING OUTWARD

Seated Upward Hands Pose

- Inhale as you reach your arms overhead and bring your palms together.

- Plant your feet hip-distance apart and let your knees come together.

- Lift your arms, interlace your fingers, and point your index fingers toward the ceiling.

- Lengthen your spine and gaze toward your hands, if it feels comfortable.

- Continue pressing through the soles of your feet, and breathe as you hold the pose

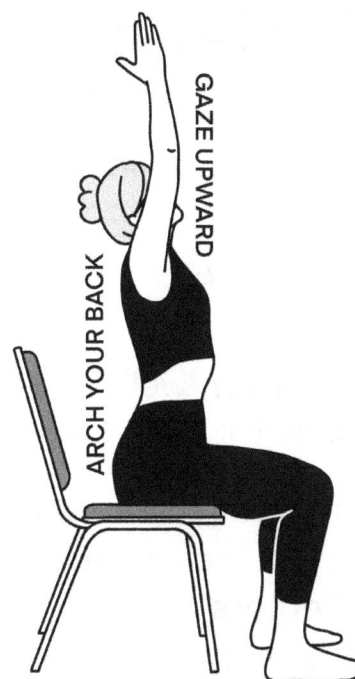

Seated Side Bend Pose

- While in seated Upward Hands Pose, exhale and extend to the right.

- Keep your feet pressed into the floor, and you feel the stretch in the left side of the body.

- Inhale back to center, release your arms, and repeat on the other side.

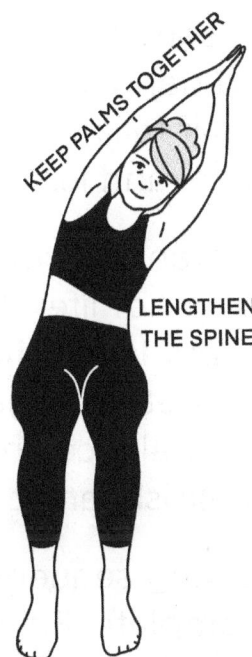

When you have completed the cycle on both sides of the body, you have finished the sequence. You can repeat the sequence as many times as you wish, if doing this as a stand-alone practice. Sun and Moon Salutations are both powerful sequences that allow us to look inward and be present. In the next chapter, we will be diving into yoga sequences for balance and flexibility.

YOGA SEQUENCES FOR BALANCE AND FLEXIBILITY

5

"You can have a plan, but you have to be flexible. Every day is unpredictable, and you just have to go with the flow."

Jane Krakowski

In this chapter, we will be focusing on yoga exercises and sequences that will target your balance and flexibility.

It's normal for the aging process to include decreased balance and flexibility. A lack of flexibility can have a serious impact on quality of life. Seniors with limited flexibility may experience posture problems, limited range of motion, a shuffled walk, a reduced walking speed, and less walking in general.

Similarly, seniors with reduced balance may experience an increased danger of falling, as well as an increased chance of injuries if falling occurs, reduced quality of life, a loss of confidence, and less social interactions.

It is important to work on balance and flexibility to maintain a good quality of life. Research has shown that **yoga improves balance and lower limb flexibility** in adults over 60 years of age. Even better, yoga has been proven to be more effective at improving balance and flexibility than walking and chair aerobics (Sivaramakrishnan et al., 2019).

The following sequences are designed to take fifteen minutes or less to complete. Each sequence blends flexibility and balance poses, and they can be completed as a stand-alone practice, or combined with the other sequences found in this guide.

EXERCISES TO IMPROVE BALANCE AND FLEXIBILITY

SEQUENCE 1: BALANCE AND HIP OPENER

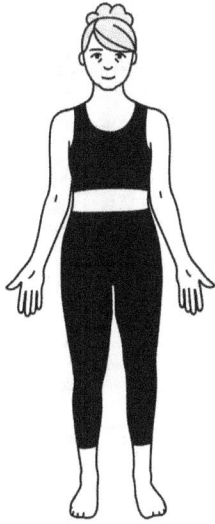

MOUNTAIN POSE

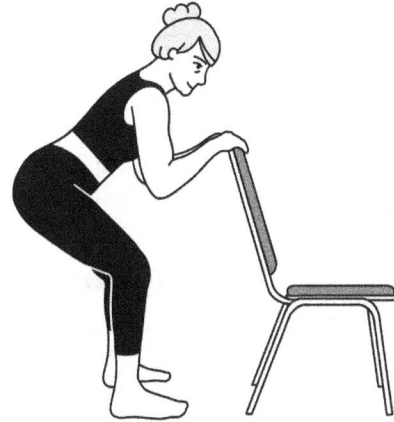

ASSISTED CHAIR POSE

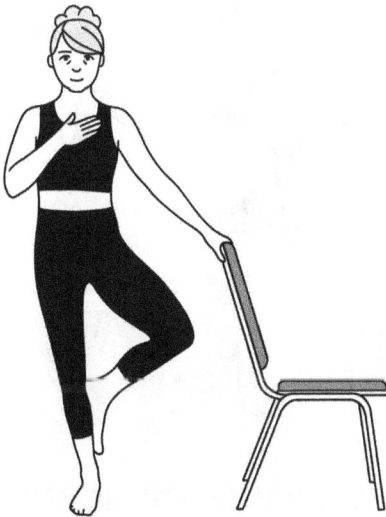

ASSISTED TREE POSE

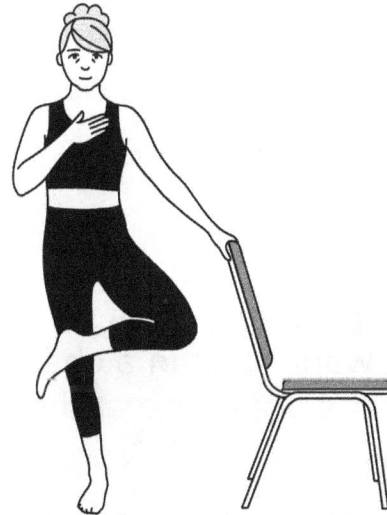

ASSISTED PIGEON POSE

Mountain Pose

- Stand in front of a chair that is propped securely against a wall.

- Place your feet hip-distance apart, press the soles of your feet into the floor, and lengthen up through the spine.

- Relax your arms by your side with palms facing forward.

- Inhale and exhale a few times to ground yourself.

KEEP CHEST OPEN

FEET ANCHORED

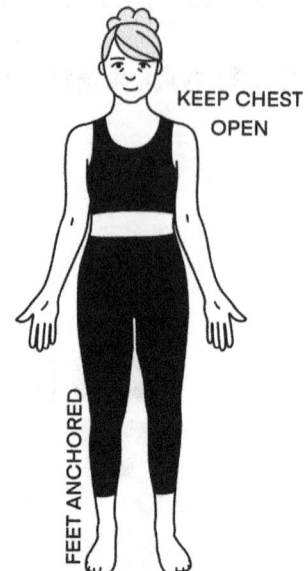

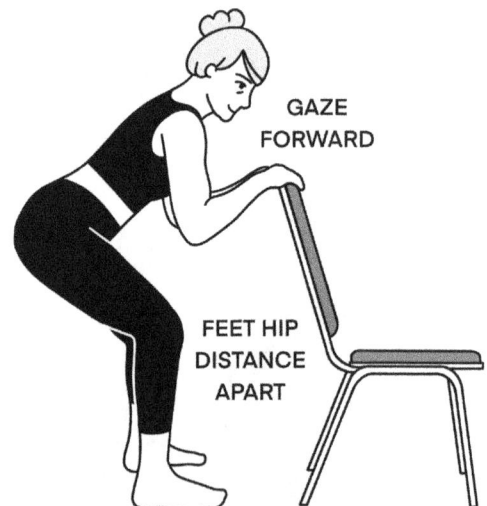

SUGGESTED MODIFICATIONS

To **decrease the challenge**, you can do this pose seated in the chair.

Assisted Chair Pose

- Inhale and bring your hands to the back of the chair.

- Exhale and slowly bend your knees.

- Lower your buttocks toward the floor, as if you want to sit in a chair. Engage your core and lift your chest.

- Keep your spine straight and your neck aligned.

- Gaze softly forward and hold the position for 3-5 breaths.

- Straighten your legs to return to standing.

GAZE FORWARD

FEET HIP DISTANCE APART

SUGGESTED MODIFICATIONS

To **decrease the challenge**, you can take the Chair Pose sitting on the chair. Your feet should still be hip-distance apart and pressing into the floor. Your arms will come up by your ears parallel to each other with the palms facing inwards. Try to lift your buttocks from the chair, if possible.

Assisted Tree Pose

- Hold onto the chair with both hands, then inhale as you shift your weight onto your right foot.

- Place your left foot on your inner right calf or on your inner right thigh, whichever is most comfortable.

- Engage your core and lengthen through your spine.

- Focus your gaze straight forward, and hold the pose for a few breaths as you try to maintain your balance on the right leg.

- Release your leg and return to standing.

- Repeat the same thing on the other side.

ENGAGE CORE

GAZE FORWARD

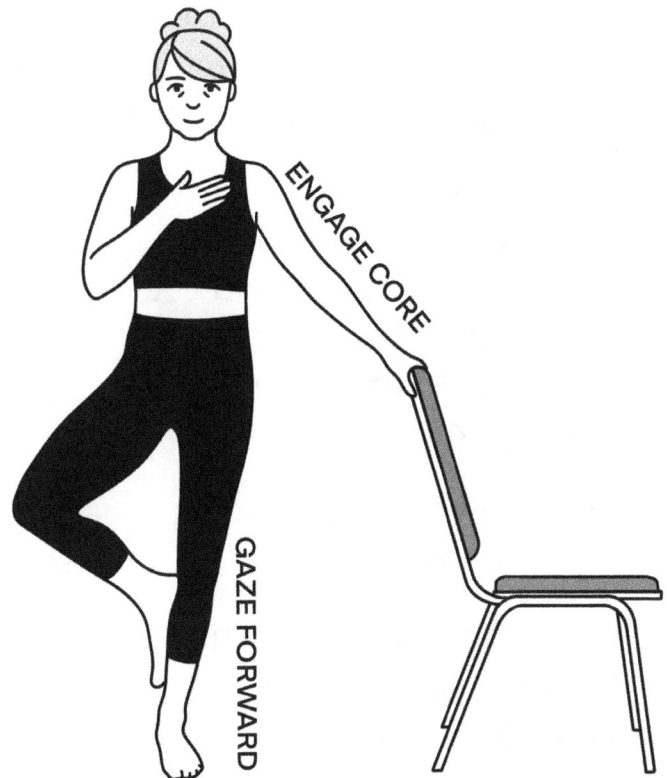

SUGGESTED MODIFICATIONS

To **decrease the challenge**, do this pose while sitting on the chair. Press one foot into the floor to anchor your leg. Open your other leg out to the side as you rest your foot on a block. The palms come together at the heart center. To **increase the challenge** in the standing Tree Pose, hold onto the back of the chair with only one hand and place the other hand at your heart center.

Assisted Pigeon Pose

- Hold onto the chair with both hands, then inhale and shift your weight onto your right foot.

- Place your left leg on top of your right thigh and flex your left foot; your legs should look like the number 4.

- Engage your core and lengthen your spine.

- Focus your gaze straight forward to help with balance.

- Hold the pose and breathe for a few moments.

- Repeat the same thing on the opposite leg.

LENGTHEN THE SPINE

HOLD THE POSE

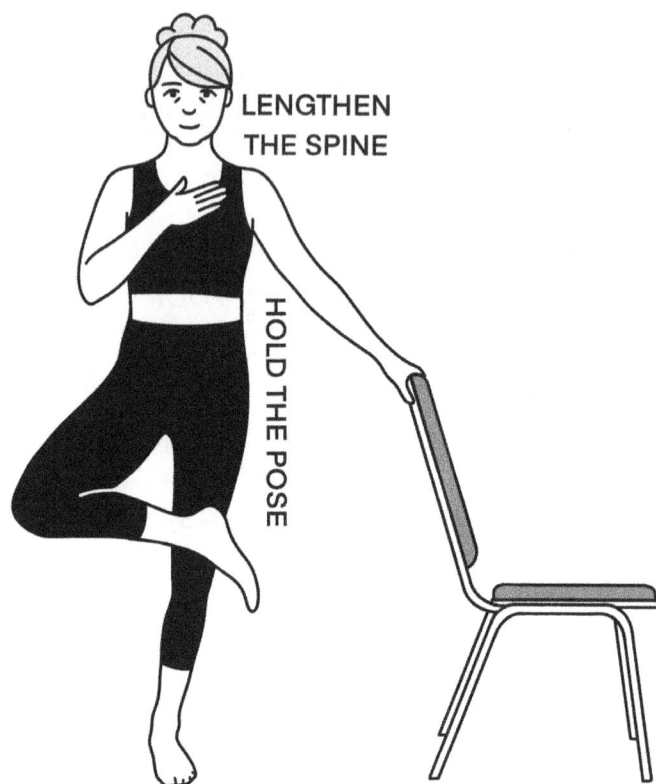

SUGGESTED MODIFICATIONS

To **decrease the challenge**, do this pose while sitting on the chair. Press one foot into the floor to anchor the leg. Bring the other foot up and press it into the anchored leg to create the shape of a number 4. The lower part of the leg is resting on the opposite thigh. Rest your hands on your hips. To **increase the challenge** from the seated variation, press gently on the bent knee to increase the stretch in your hip, or lean your torso forward.

EXERCISES TO IMPROVE BALANCE AND FLEXIBILITY

SEQUENCE 2: POSTERIOR FLEXIBILITY AND BALANCE

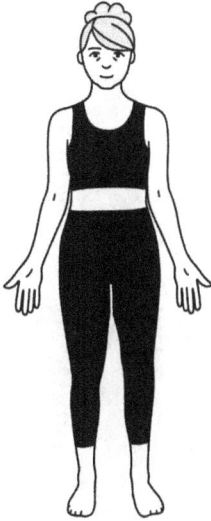

MOUNTAIN POSE

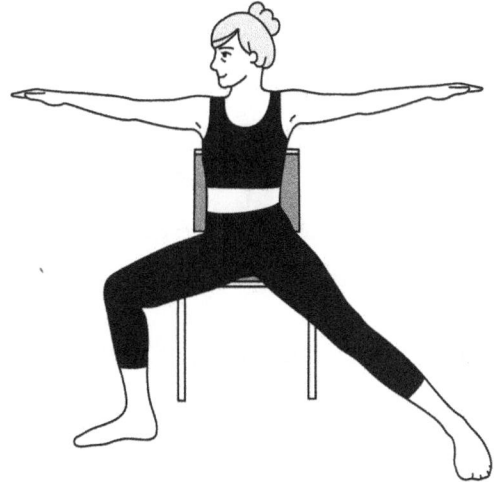

SEATED WARRIOR II POSE

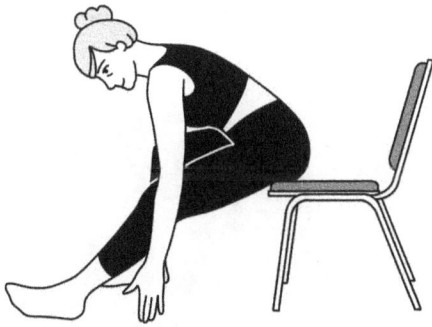

SEATED PYRAMID POSE

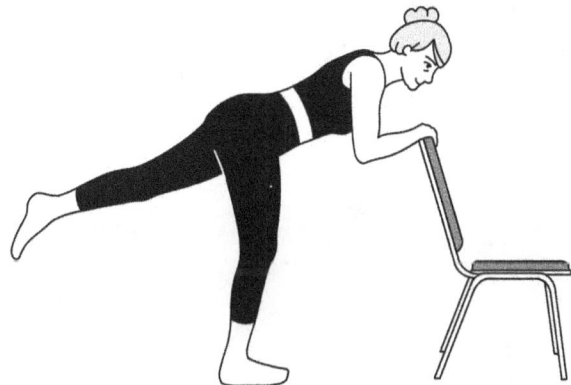

ASSISTED WARRIOR III POSE

Mountain Pose

- Begin standing with your back straight in front of a chair that is propped securely against a wall.

- Place your feet hip-distance apart, and press the soles of your feet into the ground. (Feel "all four corners" of your feet pressing firmly down).

- Your arms should be relaxed by your side with palms facing forward.

- Inhale and exhale a few times to ground yourself.

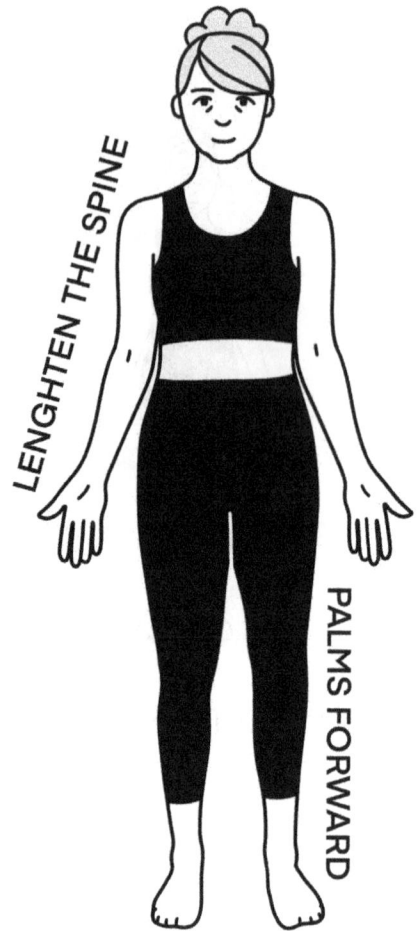

SUGGESTED MODIFICATIONS

To **decrease the challenge**, do this pose seated in the chair.

LENGHTEN THE SPINE

PALMS FORWARD

Seated Warrior II Pose

- Sit on your chair, lengthen your spine, and place your feet hip-distance apart.

- Open your right knee out to the side and point your toes to the right.

- Your right knee should be bent at about 90 degrees.

- Stretch your left leg back to form a straight line.

- Point your left toes forward.

- Extend your arms out to the sides at shoulder height, palms facing down.

- Turn your head to the right and gaze just beyond your right hand.

- Hold the pose and breathe for a few moments.

- Repeat the same thing on the opposite side.

POINT TOES FORWARD

LENGHTEN THE SPINE

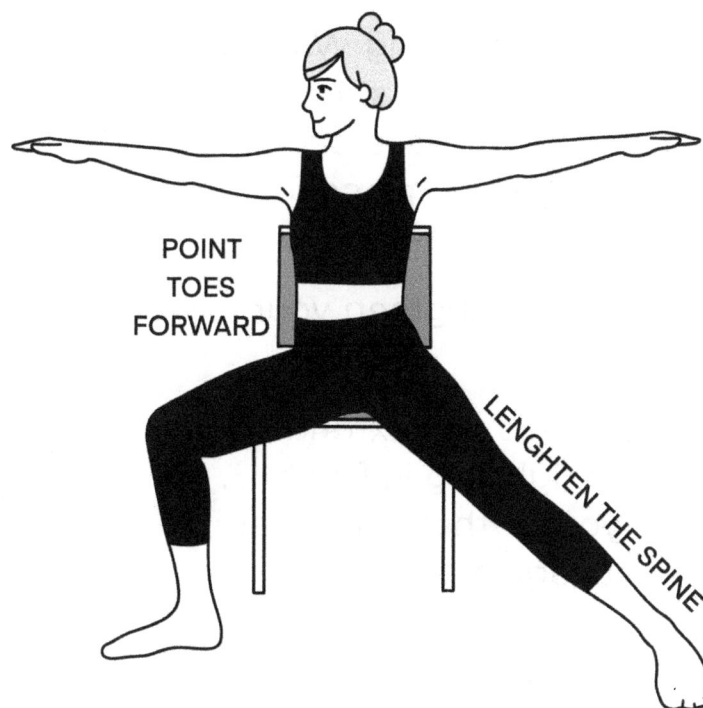

SUGGESTED MODIFICATIONS

To **decrease the challenge**, you can place your front foot on a block for support. To **increase the challenge**, you can push through your feet, lift your hips, and hover over the chair.

Seated Pyramid Pose

- After completing Warrior II Pose on both sides, bring both knees back to center and place feet hip-distance apart.

- Inhale to lengthen your spine.

- Exhale as you extend your right leg in front of you so that your heel rests against the floor.

- Hinge at the hips and fold forward while lengthening through your spine.

- You can keep your torso parallel to the floor, or fold deeper if it feels good.

- Rest both hands on the floor on either side of your right leg, and direct your gaze toward the floor.

- Hold the pose and breathe for a few moments, then repeat on the opposite side.

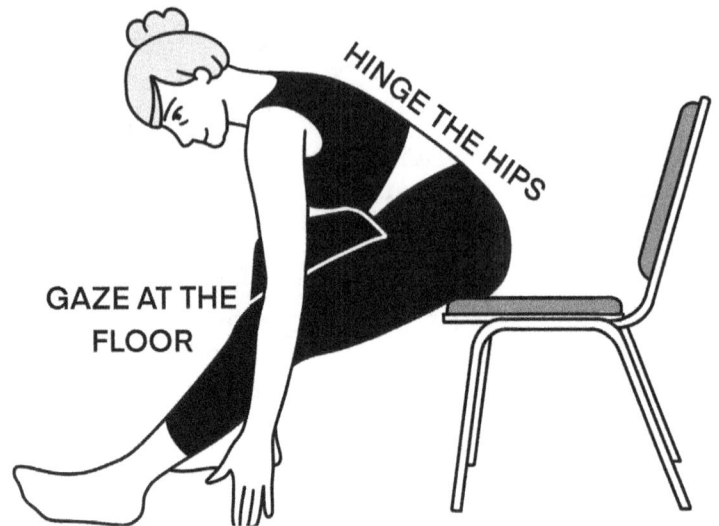

HINGE THE HIPS

GAZE AT THE FLOOR

SUGGESTED MODIFICATIONS

To **decrease the challenge**, place your hands on your shin or on your thigh instead of on the floor. For extra support, you can also rest your hands on yoga blocks on either side of your foot.

Assisted Warrior III Pose

- Return to a standing position, turn the chair and prop the seat against the wall so you are facing the back of the chair.

- Hold onto the back of the chair with both hands.

- Inhale to lengthen your spine.

- On your next exhale, transfer your weight to the right leg and hinge forward.

- Keep your right leg as straight as you can without overstraining.

- Lift your left leg behind you.

- Keep your neck aligned with the rest of your spine.

- Engage your core and press into the right foot.

- Softly gaze forward and hold the pose for a few breaths, then repeat on the other side.

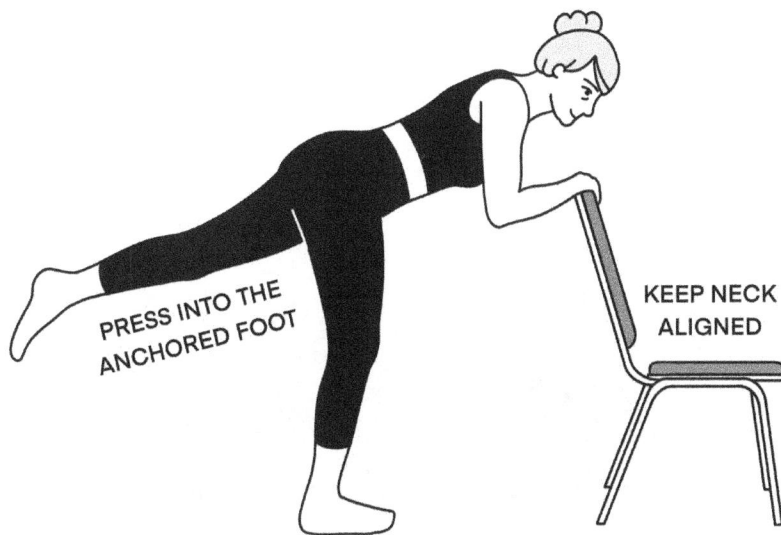

PRESS INTO THE ANCHORED FOOT

KEEP NECK ALIGNED

SUGGESTED MODIFICATIONS

To **increase the challenge**, hold onto the chair with only one hand. The other arm reaches forward toward the wall. To **decrease the challenge**, don't hinge as far forward.

EXERCISES TO IMPROVE BALANCE AND FLEXIBILITY

SEQUENCE 3: BACK OPENER AND BALANCE

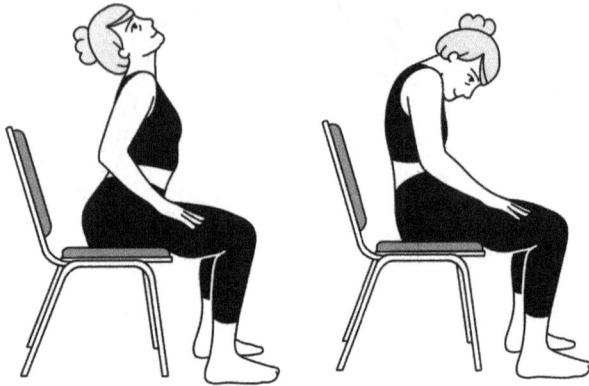

SEATED CAT AND COW POSE

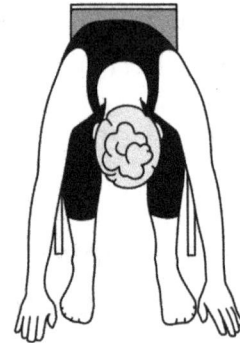

SEATED FORWARD FOLD

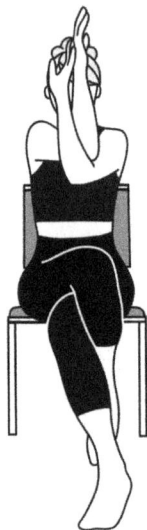

SEATED EAGLE POSE

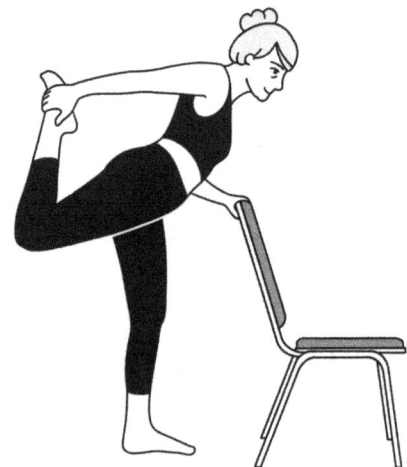

ASSISTED DANCER POSE

Seated Cat and Cow Pose

- Sit tall in a chair with your feet hip-distance apart.

- Rest both hands on your thighs.

- Inhale as you arch your back and lift your sternum toward the ceiling for Cow Pose.

- Exhale as you round your back and bring your chin toward your chest for Cat Pose.

- Alternate between these two positions while syncing your movement to your breath.

- Repeat for a few breaths.

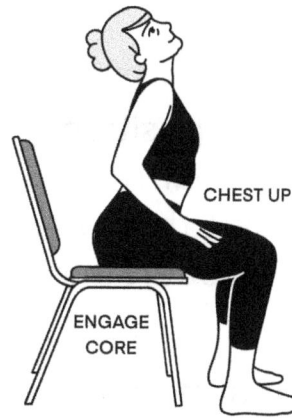

CHEST UP

ENGAGE CORE

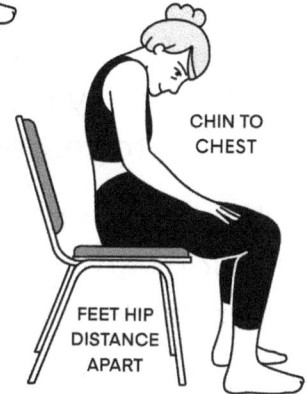

CHIN TO CHEST

FEET HIP DISTANCE APART

Seated Forward Fold

- Return to a neutral spine and keep your feet hip-distance apart.

- Inhale as you lengthen your spine.

- Exhale as you fold forward over your thighs, hinging from the hips.

- Touch the ground with your fingertips, or rest them on your thighs, whichever is more comfortable.

- Relax your shoulders, and let your head be heavy.

- Hold the pose for a few moments and breathe.

- Inhale as you return to a tall, seated position.

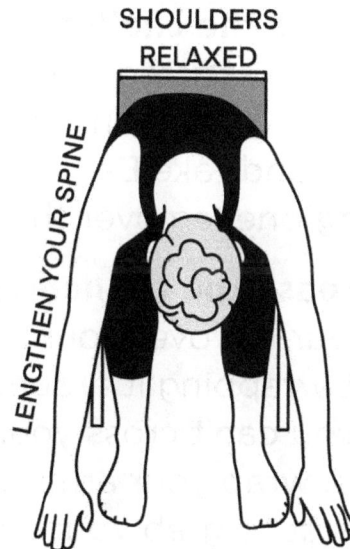

SHOULDERS RELAXED

LENGTHEN YOUR SPINE

Seated Eagle Pose

- From a tall, seated position, exhale and cross your right thigh over your left thigh and wrap your right foot around your left calf.

- Cross your right arm under your left arm and bend your elbows, trying to touch your palms together.

- Keep your elbows at shoulder height and imagine sliding forward on your rib cage.

- Feel the stretch between your shoulder blades as you hold the pose for a few breaths.

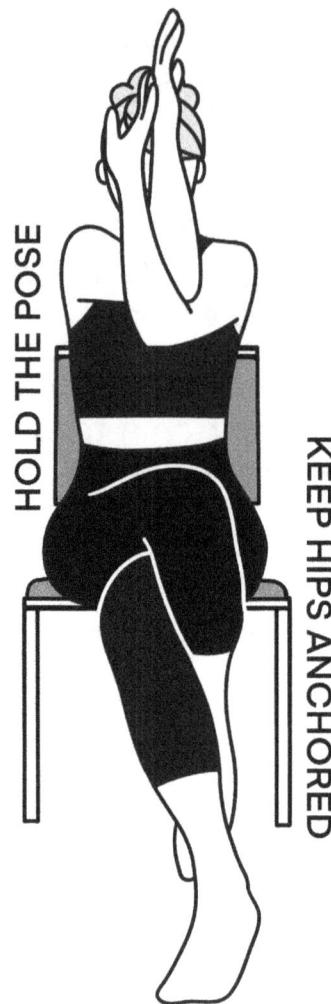

SUGGESTED MODIFICATIONS

To **increase the challenge**, you can take an assisted Eagle Pose in a standing position. Hold onto the chair and take Eagle legs (crossing one leg over the other).

To **decrease the challenge**, cross your leg over your thigh without wrapping it around the calf. If you can't cross your arms in Eagle, wrap your arms around your chest to grab your shoulder blades on either side.

HOLD THE POSE

KEEP HIPS ANCHORED

Assisted Dancer Pose

- Place the seat of the chair against the wall.

- While standing, hold onto the back of the chair with both hands, then inhale to lengthen your spine.

- Exhale as you transfer your weight to your right foot and bend your right knee.

- Bring your right hand to the inside of your right foot and hold onto it.

- Extend your right thigh backward, then lift your chest and gaze forward.

- Balance by pressing through the sole of your right foot.

- Breathe and hold the pose for a few breaths, and then repeat on the other side.

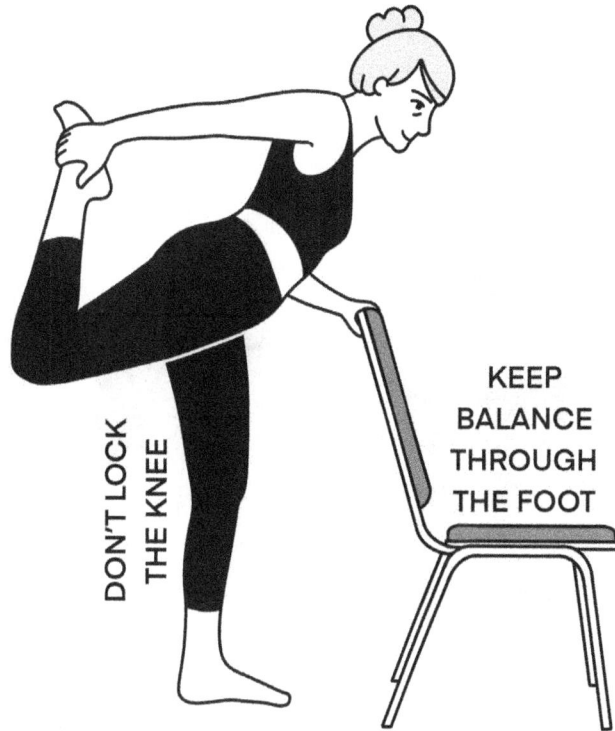

DON'T LOCK THE KNEE

KEEP BALANCE THROUGH THE FOOT

SUGGESTED MODIFICATIONS

To **decrease the challenge**, wrap a yoga strap around the ankle to support your bent leg. You can also reduce your range of motion when you bend your knee. To **increase the challenge**, lean your torso forward as you extend your leg further back to increase the stretch in the thigh.

EXERCISES TO IMPROVE BALANCE AND FLEXIBILITY

SEQUENCE 4: BACKBEND AND BALANCE

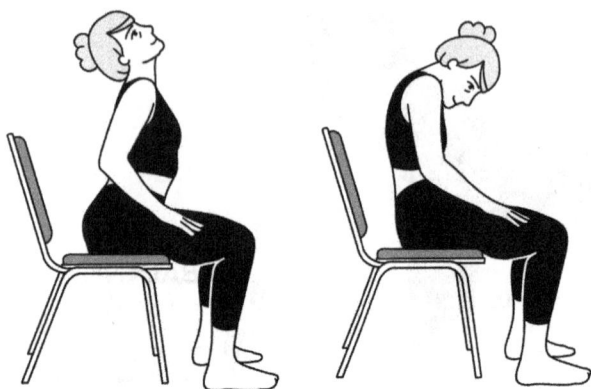

SEATED CAT AND COW POSE

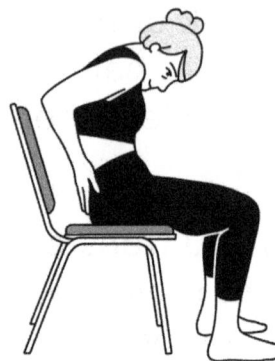

SEATED CAMEL POSE

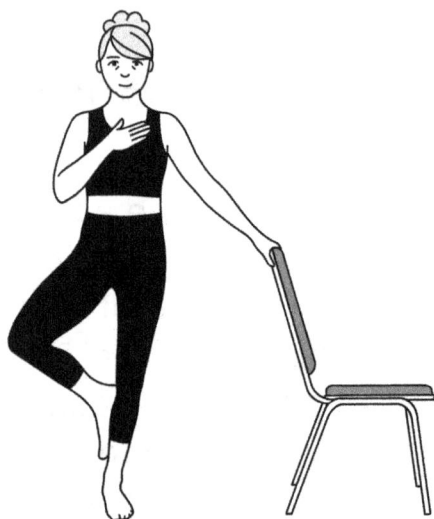

ASSISTED TREE POSE

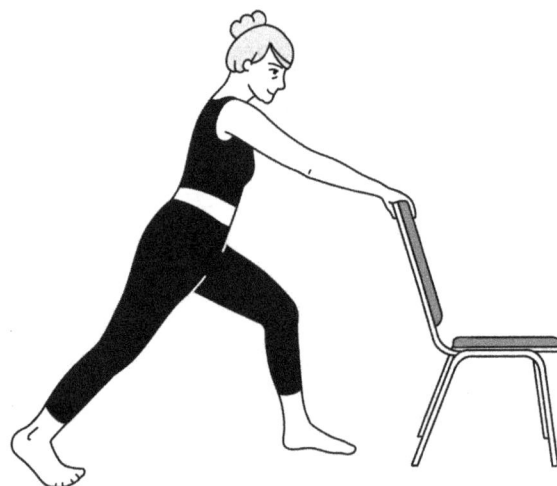

ASSISTED HIGH LUNGE POSE

Seated Cat and Cow Pose

- Sit in a chair, lengthen your spine, and place your feet hip-distance apart.

- Rest both hands on your thighs.

- Inhale as you arch your back and lift your sternum toward the ceiling for Cow Pose.

- Exhale as you round your back and bring your chin toward your chest for Cat Pose.

- Alternate between these two positions while syncing your movement to your breath.

- Repeat for a few breaths, then return to a neutral spine.

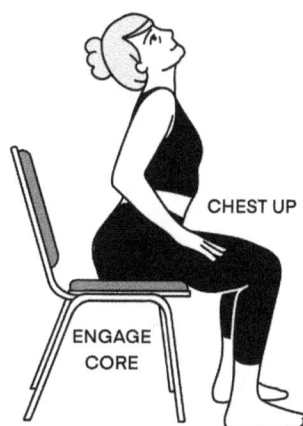

CHEST UP

ENGAGE CORE

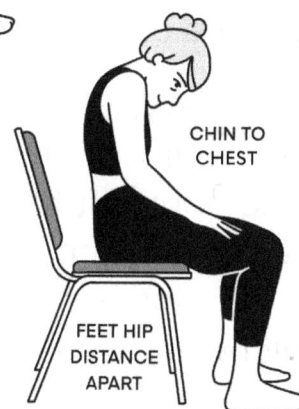

CHIN TO CHEST

FEET HIP DISTANCE APART

Seated Camel Pose

- Inhale, lift your chest, and lengthen your spine.

- Bring your hands to your lower back and point your fingertips toward the floor.

- Exhale and slowly arch your back while tucking your chin.

- Breathe and hold the pose for a few moments. On every inhale, expand your ribcage. On every exhale, try to arch your back a little more.

- Return to an upright seated position.

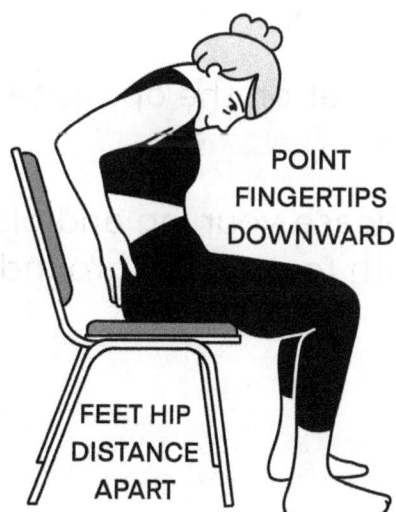

POINT FINGERTIPS DOWNWARD

FEET HIP DISTANCE APART

Assisted Tree Pose

- Stand up and prop the chair with the seat against the wall.

- Hold onto the back of the chair with both hands, and stand tall with feet hip-distance apart.

- Inhale, shift your weight onto your right foot, and place your left foot on your inner right calf or on your inner right thigh, whichever feels best.

- Engage your core, lengthen your spine, and gaze straight ahead.

- Breathe and hold the pose for a few moments as you try to maintain your balance.

- Repeat on the opposite side.

- Release your leg and place both feet on the ground.

MAINTAIN YOUR BALANCE

MIND YOUR BREATH

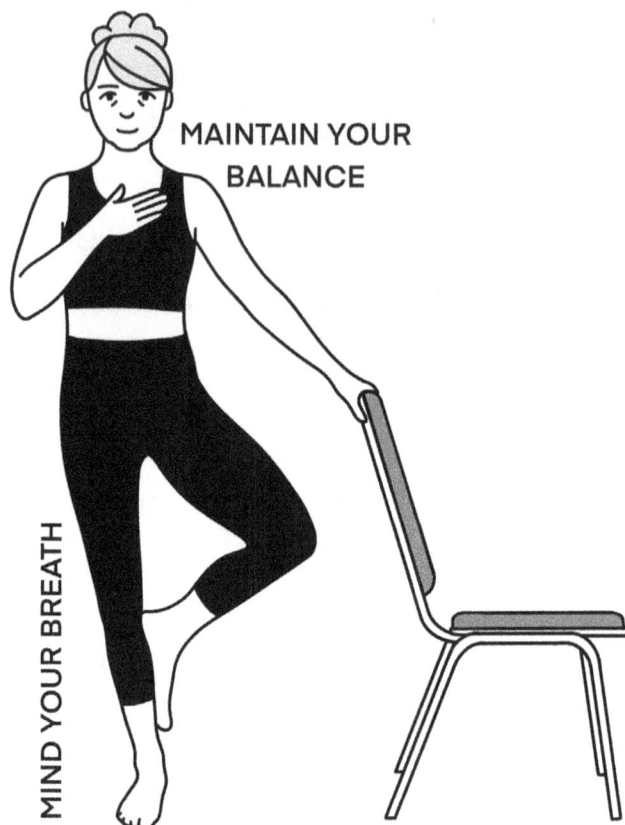

SUGGESTED MODIFICATIONS

To **decrease the challenge**, sit on the chair while performing this pose. Keep one foot pressing into the ground. Rest your other foot on a block and open the leg out to the side. Press your palms together at the heart center. To **increase the challenge**, in the standing Tree Pose, hold onto the back of the chair with one hand, and place your other hand at your heart center.

Assisted High Lunge Pose

- Inhale, lengthen your spine, and hold onto the back of the chair.

- Exhale, step your right foot back, lift your right heel, and stand on the ball of your right foot.

- Keep the right knee straight but not locked.

- Anchor the left foot by pressing through the sole of the foot. Engage the left knee so that it doesn't sink toward the midline.

- Lengthen your spine, engage your core, gaze softly forward, and hold the pose for a few moments.

- Repeat on the other side.

TOES POINTING FORWARD

KEEP NECK ALIGNED

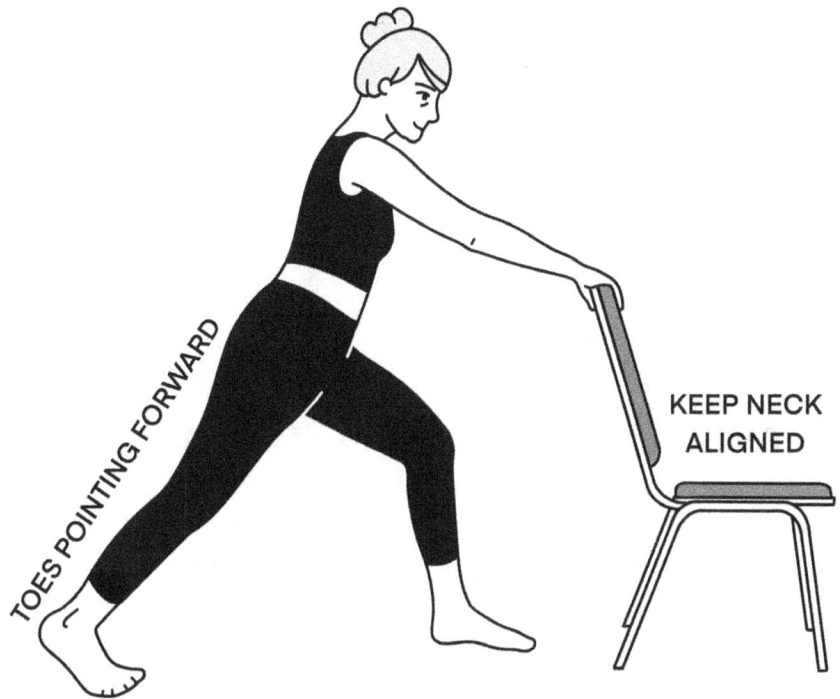

SUGGESTED MODIFICATIONS

To **increase the challenge**, raise one arm overhead. To **decrease the challenge**, reduce how wide your stance is, so that you are standing with your feet closer together.

HOW TO INCORPORATE MINDFULNESS TECHNIQUES

As you continue to practice all of these different sequences, it's important you remember to integrate mindfulness into your movement. Simply put, mindfulness is being fully present and living in the moment, without any distractions or judgment. Being mindful is easier said than done, and that's why mindfulness is something we practice. We come back to it repeatedly, and with time, we get better at it.

Here are a few tips to help you be mindful throughout your yoga practice:

1. CHECK IN WITH YOUR FEELINGS

Notice how you're feeling before, during, and after a yoga practice. The goal is not to judge how you feel, but simply to notice or to observe. By noticing how you feel, you can adapt your practice to better suit your needs. For example, if you woke up with a sore lower back, consider being gentle with yourself and don't go as deep in your backbends. You may notice that your energy changes throughout your practice; pay attention to the subtle changes in your mind and body.

2. LET GO OF EXPECTATIONS

Sometimes, you may notice that you have expectations for how or what you should be doing in a pose. You might find yourself thinking, "Why can't I touch the floor?" or "I wish my legs weren't so tight!" Pay attention to those expectations, and then choose to be kind with yourself instead. If you are harsh with yourself, you miss an opportunity to practice mindfulness.

Let go of your expectations for the yoga session and meet your body where it is each day. Modify a pose or use props, so that your body feels good.

3. REFOCUS YOUR ATTENTION

Whenever you feel like your thoughts are racing, whether that is thinking about your day ahead or something that worries you, try to return your attention to the present moment. Bring your attention to the here and now.

For example, if you're in a pose, you may notice that you're not focused, and that it's difficult to balance. As soon as you realize you have stopped being mindful, take a moment to acknowledge the distraction, and refocus your attention on your body. To do this, focus on your breath, notice how your body feels, and bring your awareness to your body's position in space.

Remember that a mindful practice, like a yoga practice, is a constant work in progress. In the next chapter, we will be diving into different yoga sequences to improve cardiovascular fitness.

YOGA SEQUENCES FOR CARDIOVASCULAR HEALTH

6

"The best and most beautiful things in the world cannot be seen or even touched—they must be felt with the heart."

Hellen Keller

In this chapter, you'll learn yoga sequences to improve heart health. According to the World Health Organization, an estimated 17.9 million deaths are caused by heart disease each year. Many risk factors can be associated with heart disease:

- High blood pressure (hypertension)
- High cholesterol
- Smoking
- Diabetes
- Obesity
- Unhealthy diet
- Physical inactivity
- Excessive alcohol consumption

Maintaining a good diet is one of the best ways to limit these risk factors; we will discuss this further in a later chapter. It is also important to take part in regular physical activity. The American Heart Association recommends at least 150 minutes of moderate-intensity aerobic activity or 75 minutes of vigorous-intensity aerobic activity (or a combination of both) for adults every week.

Yoga can be a beneficial way to increase your weekly aerobic activity. A recent study found that yoga can help reduce high blood pressure, improve body composition, blood glucose levels, and blood lipids (Isath et al., 2023).

To support heart health, practice yoga sequences that increase heart rate for aerobic fitness, as well as yoga sequences that slow down heart rate and reduce blood pressure. Additionally, if you practice linking breath and movement during yoga, you can bring more mindfulness into your practice, and consequently experience more mindful stress reduction on a day-to-day basis.

Before you begin, check with your physician, if you haven't done so already. Regular health check-ups and screenings usually include blood tests, blood pressure checks, cholesterol tests, and diabetes screenings. These screenings can help detect and manage risk factors that can lead to cardiovascular problems.

Below you will find three yoga sequences for heart health. Sequences one and two aim to increase the heart rate, while sequence three is meant to reduce heart rate and, consequently, reduce stress.

LOW-IMPACT CARDIO EXERCISES TO IMPROVE HEART HEALTH

SEQUENCE 1: CHAIR WARRIOR FLOW

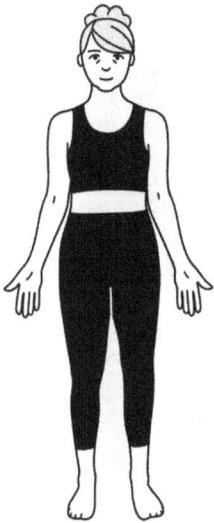

MOUNTAIN POSE

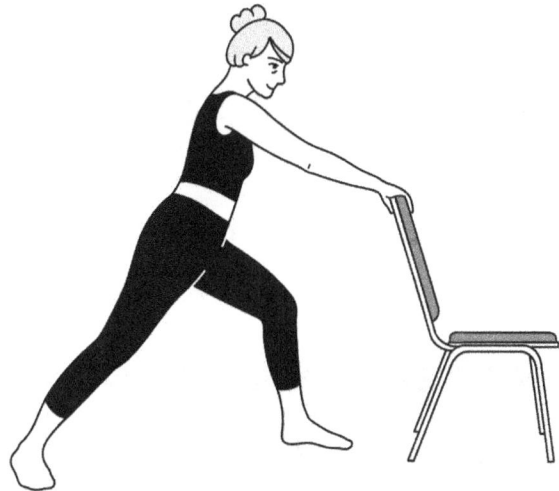

ASSISTED WARRIOR I POSE

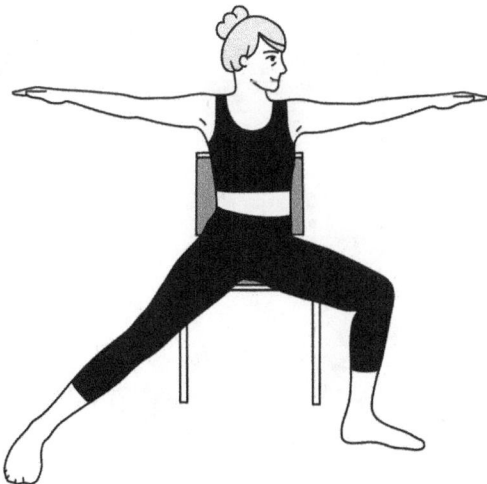

SEATED WARRIOR II POSE

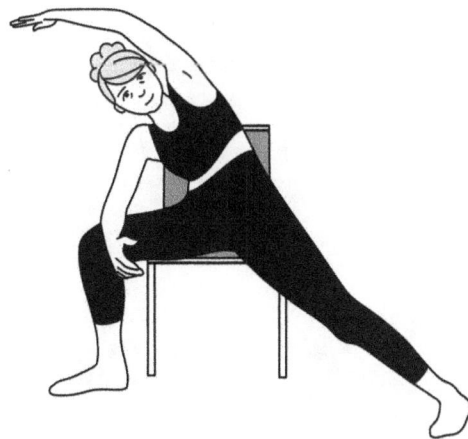

SIDE ANGLE POSE

Mountain Pose

- Stand with your back straight in front of a chair that is propped securely against a wall.

- Place your feet hip-distance apart, and press the soles of your feet into the ground. (Feel "all four corners" of your feet pressing firmly down).

- Relax your arms by your side with palms facing forward.

- Take a few breaths to ground yourself.

SUGGESTED MODIFICATIONS

To **decrease the challenge**, you can do this pose seated in the chair.

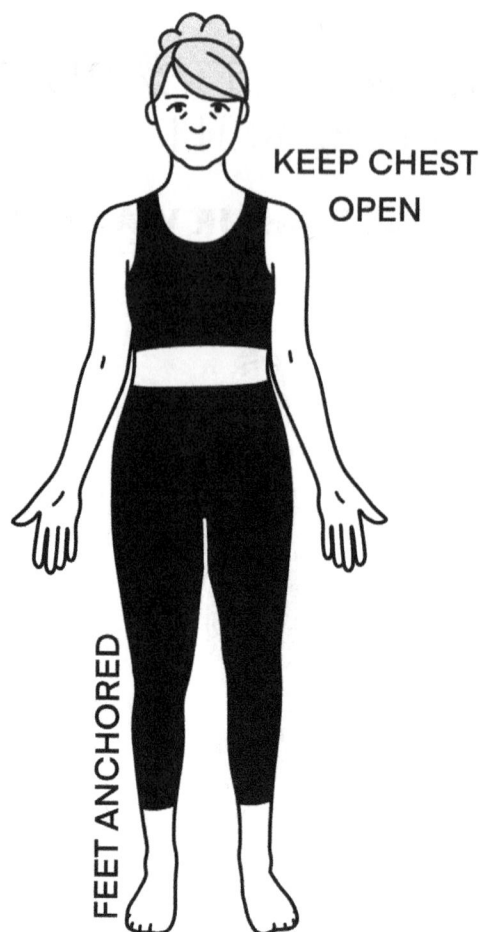

KEEP CHEST OPEN

FEET ANCHORED

Assisted Warrior I Pose

- Inhale, lengthen your spine, and hold onto the back of the chair with both hands.

- Exhale and step your right foot back into a lunge.

- Keep your left knee bent and your right leg straight.

- Turn the foot of the back leg out to a 45-degree angle.

- Hold the pose and breathe.

- On an inhale, bring both feet back together, and on the exhale, extend one leg back into Warrior I Pose.

- Alternate on each side, repeating 8-10 times while linking movement to breath in a controlled manner.

- Inhale and return to a tall upright position.

HOLD THE POSE

HOLD THE CHAIR FOR BALANCE

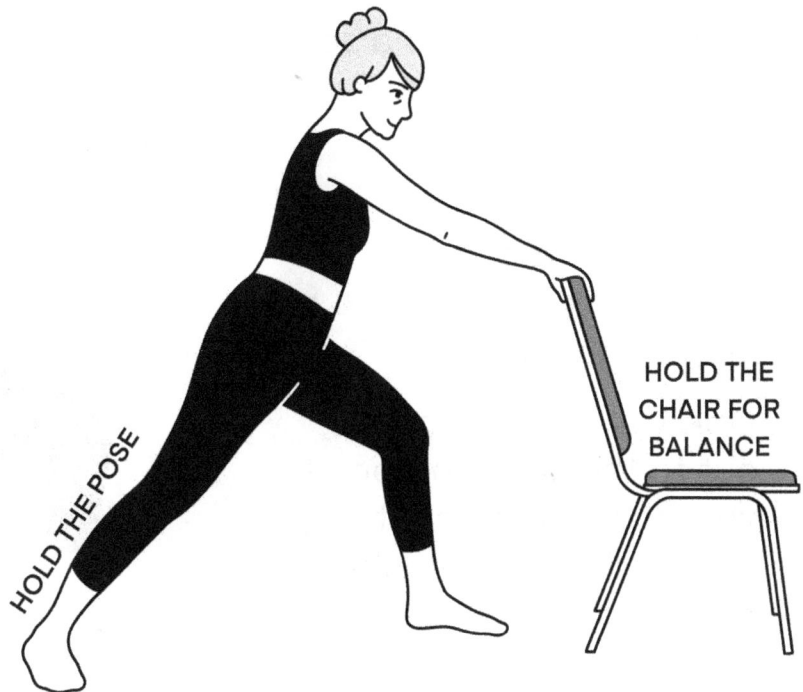

SUGGESTED MODIFICATIONS

To **increase the challenge**, hold onto the chair with only one hand. Raise your other arm overhead with the palm facing inward. To **decrease the challenge**, take a smaller step backward so that it is easier to balance.

Seated Warrior II Pose

- Turn the chair around so the back of the chair is against the wall.

- Take a seat on the chair, place your feet hip-distance apart, and lengthen your spine.

- Open your right knee out to the side, and point your toes to the right. Your right knee should be bent at about 90 degrees.

- Stretch your left leg back to form a straight line. Your left toes should point forward.

- Extend your arms out to the sides at shoulder height, palms facing down, and turn your head so you can gaze over your right hand.

- To increase your heart rate, inhale as you push through both feet and lift your hips to hover above the chair, and then exhale as you sit back down.

- Repeat 8-10 times on each side.

POINT TOES FORWARD

LENGHTEN THE SPINE

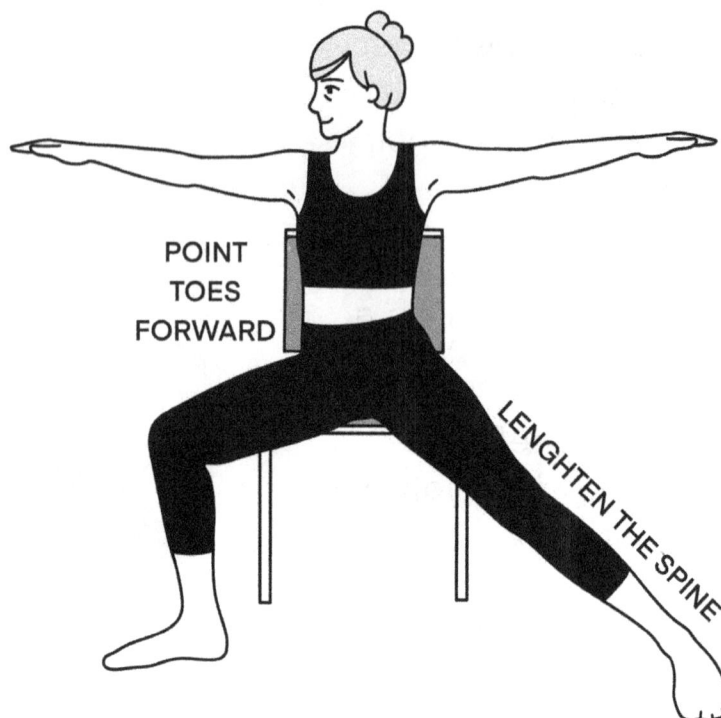

SUGGESTED MODIFICATIONS

If you can't reach the floor, you can place your front foot on a block.

Side Angle Pose

- Return to a seated position with both legs centered. Lengthen your spine and exhale as you take Warrior II legs again.

- Open your right knee out to the side and point your toes to the right. Keep your right knee bent at about 90 degrees.

- Stretch your left leg back so it forms a straight line and point your left toes forward.

- Rest your right forearm against your right thigh and extend your left arm overhead.

- Create a straight line from your left foot to your right fingertips.

- You can look up toward the ceiling, or straight ahead, whichever feels gentler on your neck.

- To increase your heart rate, keep your leg position the same, and then exhale as you lean into a side angle position, and inhale as you lift and straighten your torso. Repeat 8-10 times.

- Repeat the same exercise on the opposite side.

FEEL THE STRETCH

POINT TOES FORWARD

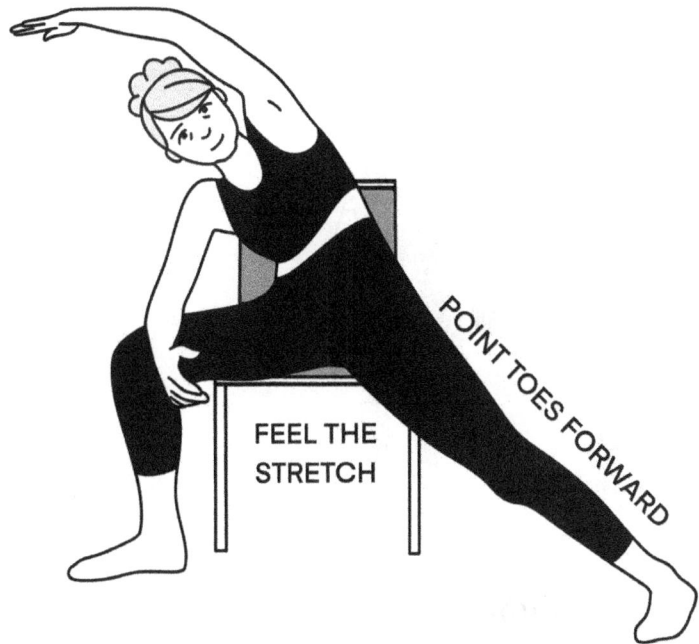

SUGGESTED MODIFICATIONS

To **decrease the challenge**, hold the extended side angle position for 8-10 breaths on each side instead of alternating between sitting upright and bending into the extended position.

LOW-IMPACT CARDIO EXERCISES TO IMPROVE HEART HEALTH

SEQUENCE 2: CHAIR POWER FLOW

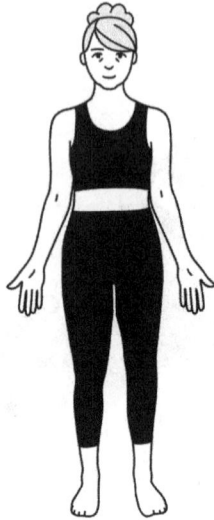

MOUNTAIN POSE

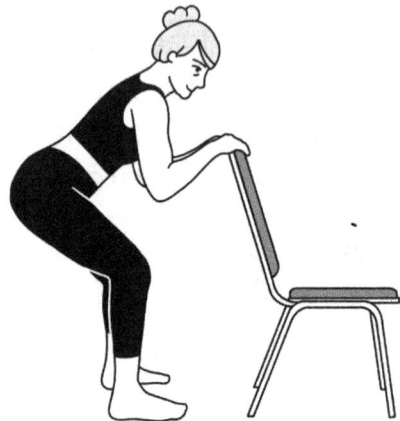

ASSISTED CHAIR POSE

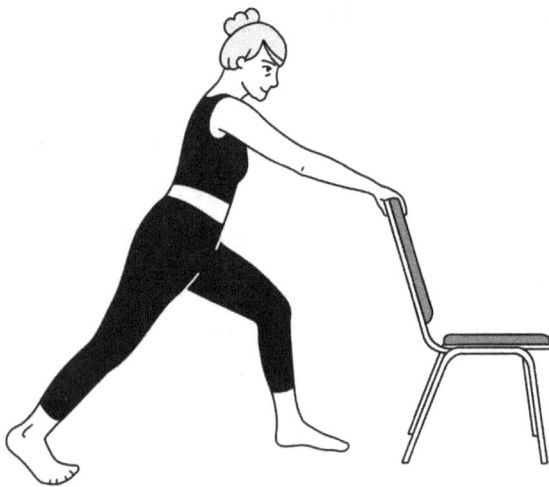

ASSISTED HIGH LUNGE POSE

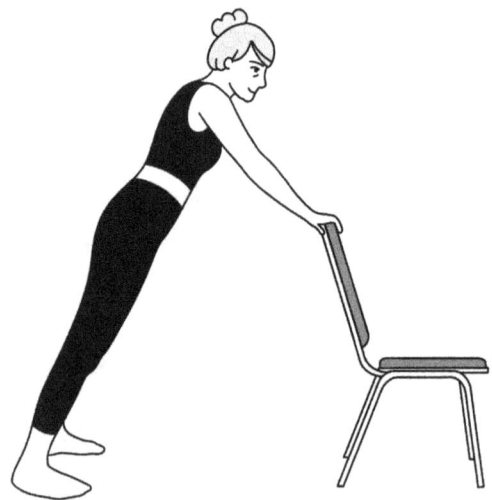

CHAIR PLANK POSE

Mountain Pose

- Stand with your back straight in front of a chair that is propped securely against a wall.

- Place your feet hip-distance apart, and press the soles of your feet into the ground. (Feel "all four corners" of your feet press firmly down).

- Relax your arms by your side with palms facing forward, and inhale and exhale a few times to ground yourself.

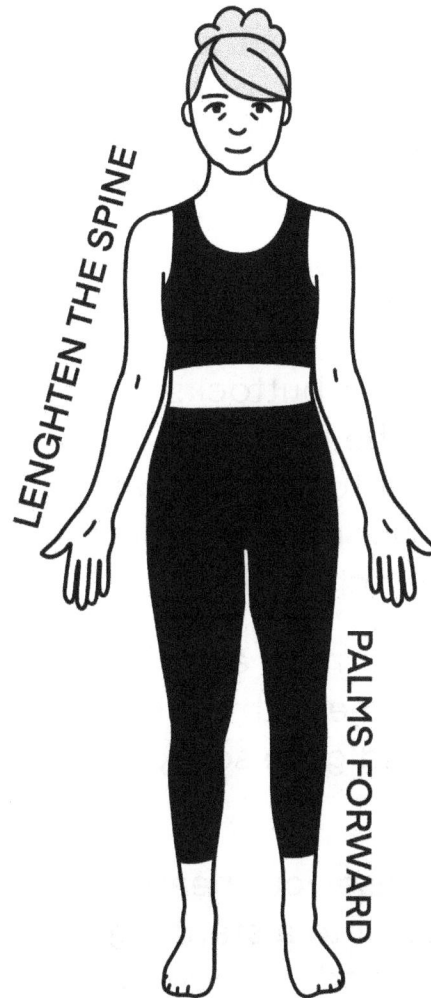

SUGGESTED MODIFICATIONS

To **decrease the challenge**, you can do this pose seated in a chair.

LENGHTEN THE SPINE

PALMS FORWARD

Assisted Chair Pose

- After a few breaths in Mountain Pose, bring your hands to the back of the chair on an inhale.

- Exhale as you bend your knees.

- Lower your buttocks toward the floor, as if you want to sit in a chair. Keep your core engaged and your chest lifted.

- Keep your neck and spine in line with each other, and gaze softly forward.

- To increase your heart rate, rise into a standing position and then lower into Chair Pose. Exhale as you bend your knees, and inhale as you straighten your knees and return to standing. Repeat 10-15 times.

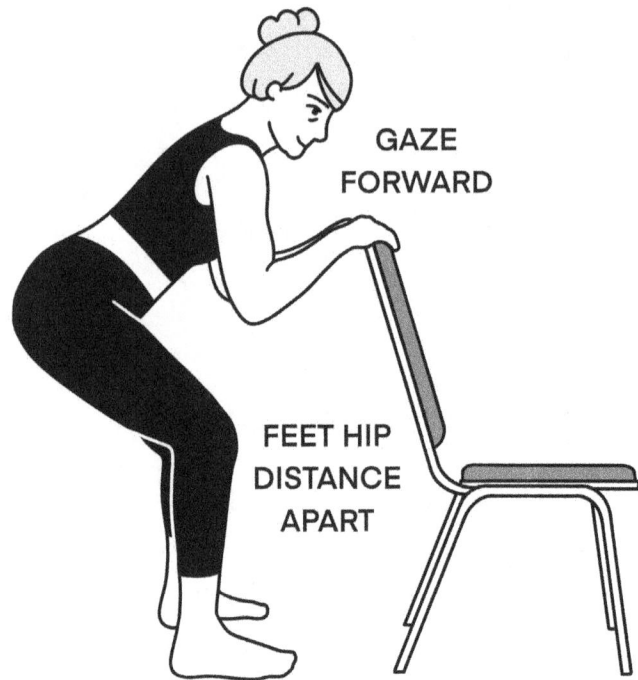

- Inhale, straighten your knees, and return to standing.

GAZE FORWARD

FEET HIP DISTANCE APART

SUGGESTED MODIFICATIONS

To **increase the challenge**, you can hold onto the back of the chair with only one hand. To **decrease the challenge**, perform the Chair Pose sitting on the chair: your feet should still be hip-distance apart and pressing into the floor. Your arms will come up by your ears parallel to each other with the palms facing inwards. Lift your buttocks from the chair and hover just above the seat.

Assisted High Lunge Pose

- Continue to hold onto the back of the chair. Exhale as you step your right foot back and stand on the ball of your right foot with your right heel lifted.

- Keep the right knee straight without locking it.

- Anchor the left foot into the ground and engage your left knee so that it doesn't fall in toward the midline.

- Gaze forward, lift your spine, and engage your core.

- To increase your heart rate, alternate between bending your front knee into High Lunge Pose on an exhale and straightening your front knee on an inhale. Repeat 8-10 times on each side.

- Inhale and return to a standing position.

ENGAGE THE KNEE

GAZE FORWARD

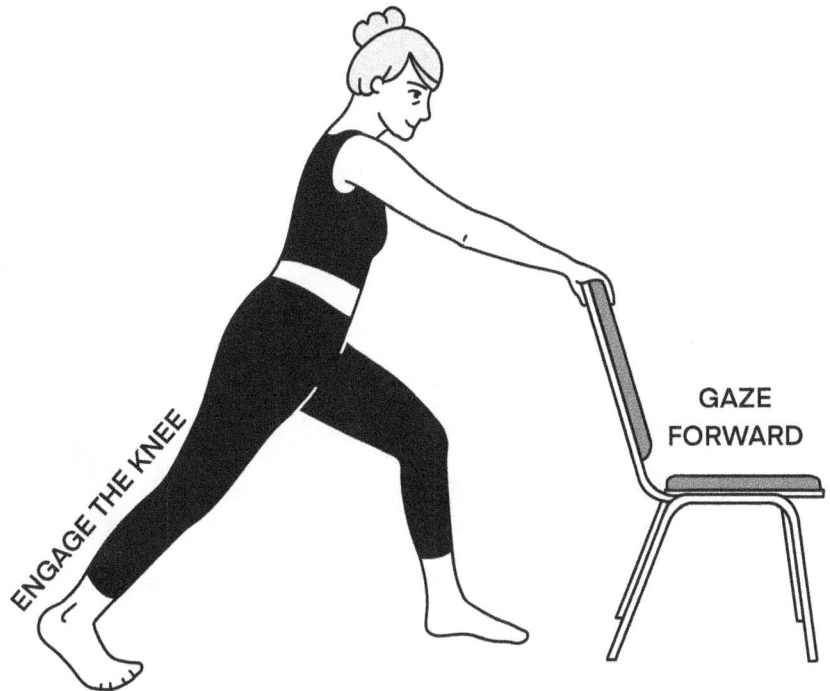

SUGGESTED MODIFICATIONS

To **increase the challenge**, release one hand from the chair and lift the arm straight overhead. To **decrease the challenge**, take a smaller step with the back leg so that you have more balance.

Chair Plank Pose

- While standing, place your hands on the seat of the chair.

- Exhale as you extend your legs back into a modified plank position.

- Keep your elbows and knees straight, but not locked.

- Position your wrists under your shoulders and keep your neck in line with the rest of your spine.

- Engage your core by pulling your navel towards your spine, and hold the position for a few breaths.

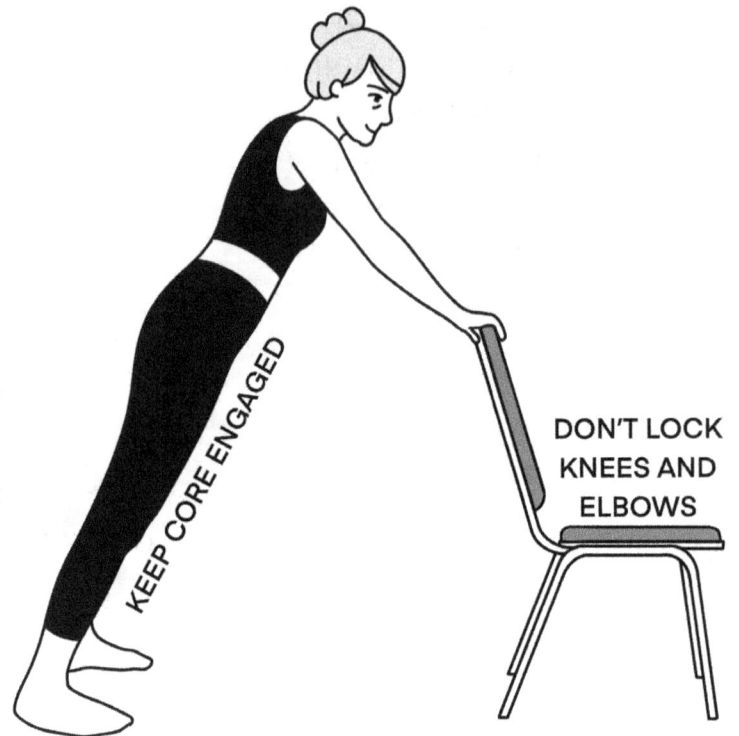

KEEP CORE ENGAGED

DON'T LOCK KNEES AND ELBOWS

SUGGESTED MODIFICATIONS

To **increase the challenge**, pull one knee towards your chest at a time, as if you're climbing a mountain. Exhale as you bring your knee toward your chest and inhale as you extend the leg out. To **decrease the challenge**, reduce the distance you step your feet back, so your body is on less of an incline.

LOW-IMPACT CARDIO EXERCISES TO IMPROVE HEART HEALTH

SEQUENCE 3: CHAIR SLOW FLOW

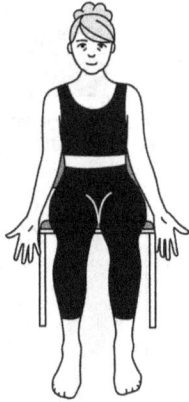

SEATED MOUNTAIN POSE

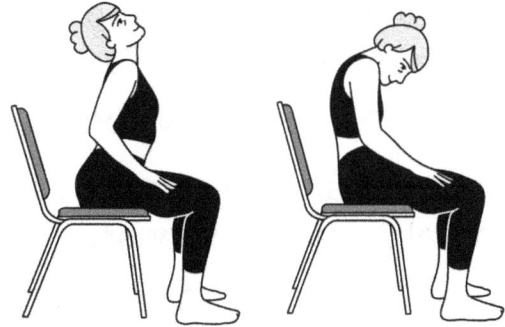

SEATED CAT AND COW POSE

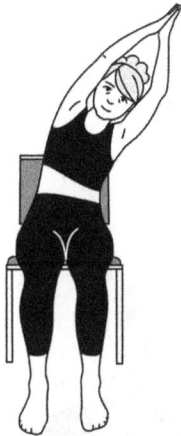

SEATED SIDE BEND POSE

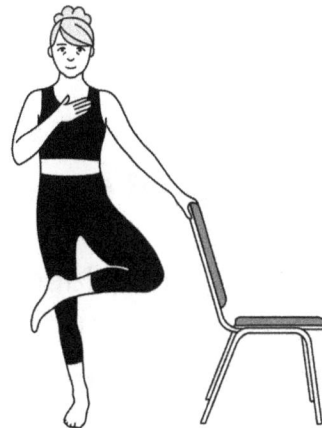

ASSISTED PIGEON POSE

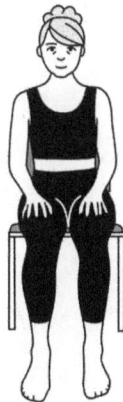

SEATED RELAXATION

Seated Mountain Pose

- Begin seated with your back straight.

- Place your feet hip-distance apart, and press the soles of your feet into the ground.

- Relax your arms by your side with palms facing forward.

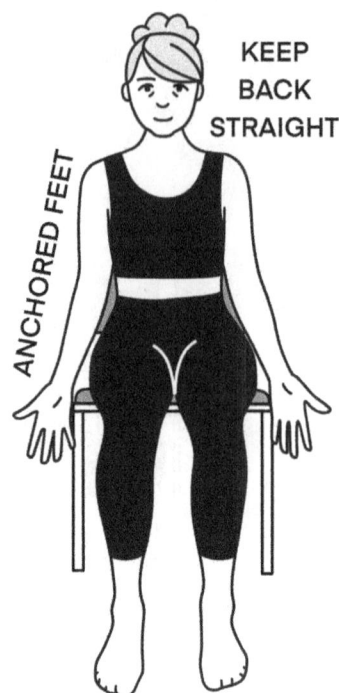

KEEP BACK STRAIGHT

ANCHORED FEET

Seated Cat and Cow Pose

- Sit tall in a chair, place your feet hip-distance apart, and rest your hands on your thighs.

- Inhale as you arch your back and lift your sternum toward the ceiling for Cow Pose.

- Exhale as you round your back and bring your chin toward your chest for Cat Pose.

- Move back and forth between Cat and Cow Pose while syncing your movement to your breath. Repeat for a few breaths.

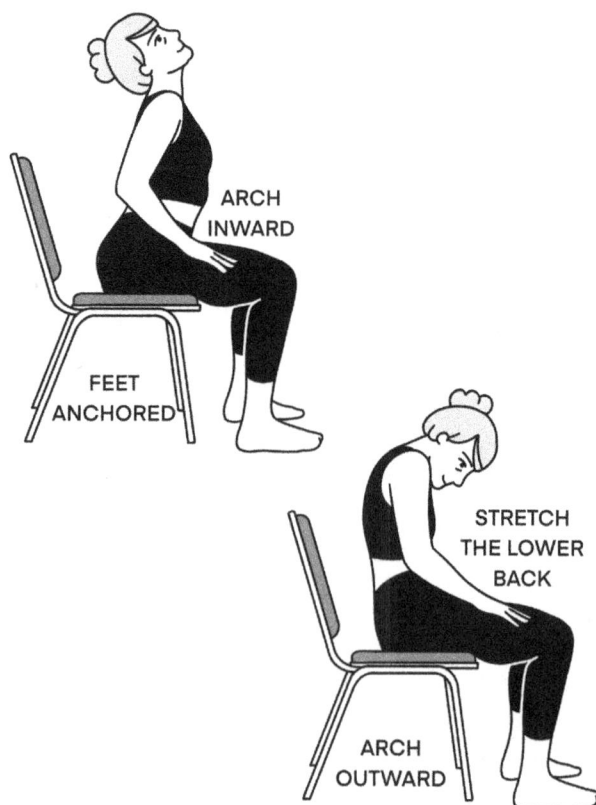

ARCH INWARD

FEET ANCHORED

STRETCH THE LOWER BACK

ARCH OUTWARD

Seated Side Bend Pose

- Inhale as you reach both arms overhead, then interlace your fingers with your thumbs and index fingers touching.

- Exhale as you extend your torso to the right.

- Press your feet into the floor, and feel the stretch in the left side of the body. Hold the position for a few breaths, then inhale back to center, and repeat the same movement on the left side.

- Inhale and return to the center, then exhale as you release your arms.

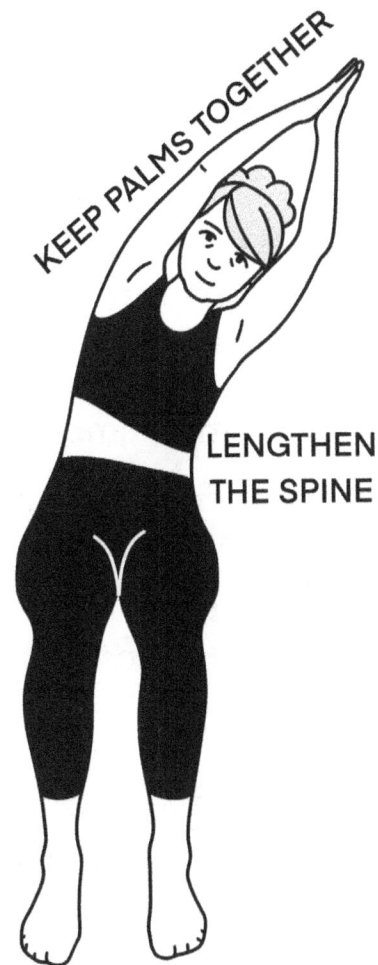

KEEP PALMS TOGETHER

LENGTHEN THE SPINE

Assisted Pigeon Pose

- In a seated position, use your hands to place your left ankle on top of your right thigh and pull the toes of your left foot toward your left shin. Your left leg should form the shape of the number 4.

- Place your hands on your hips, engage your core, and lengthen your spine.

- Gaze softly forward and hold the pose for a few breaths as you feel a stretch in the left hip.

- Repeat the same exercise on the opposite leg.

LENGTHEN THE SPINE

HOLD THE POSE

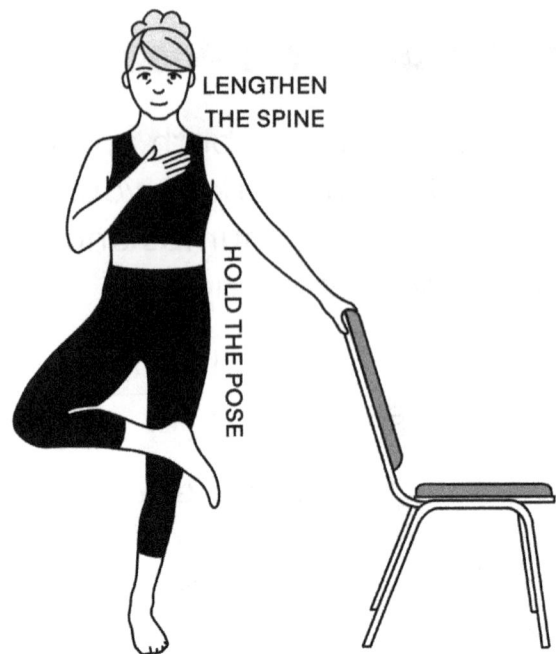

SUGGESTED MODIFICATIONS

To **increase the challenge**, gently press on the bent knee to deepen the stretch in your hip, and lean forward slightly and incline your torso.

Seated Relaxation

- Take a moment at the end of the sequence to close your eyes and focus on your breath.

- Sit tall and feel the support of the chair beneath you as you keep your feet pressed into the ground hip-distance apart. Stay in this relaxed state for a few slow, deep breaths.

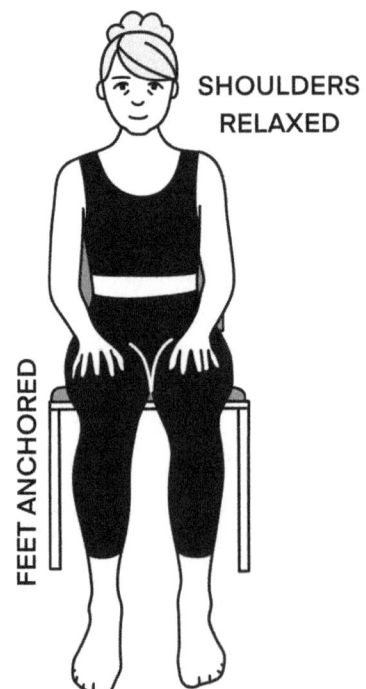

SHOULDERS RELAXED

FEET ANCHORED

YOGA SEQUENCES FOR STRENGTH-BUILDING

7

"Life doesn't get easier or more forgiving, we get stronger and more resilient."

Steve Maraboli

As we age, we naturally lose muscle mass and strength.

Both age-related and environmental factors can contribute to muscle loss. Environmental factors include less physical activity and lack of adequate nutrition (Walston, 2012). Age-related changes factors include reduced muscle mass, reduced hormones (which are important in maintaining muscle mass), and increased inflammation (Walston, 2012).

The good news is, some things can be done to positively impact some of the factors. It has been shown that focusing on physical activity and nutrition are some of the most effective ways to prevent and slow down the impact of muscle tissue loss (Volpi et al., 2004; Walston, 2012).

Yoga can also help with muscle health. A recent study highlighted that adults in their 60s and 70s who practiced yoga for 9-12 weeks had significant positive effects on physical fitness by improving muscle strength, along with balance and flexibility (Shin, 2021).

The following four yoga sequences focus on building muscle strength for the benefit of your health and well-being.

YOGA SEQUENCES FOR STRENGTH-BUILDING

SEQUENCE 1: YOGA FOR LOWER BODY STRENGTH

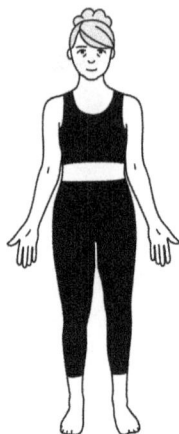

MOUNTAIN POSE

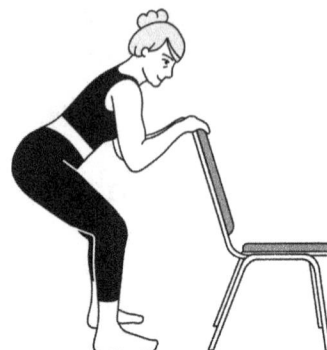

ASSISTED CHAIR POSE

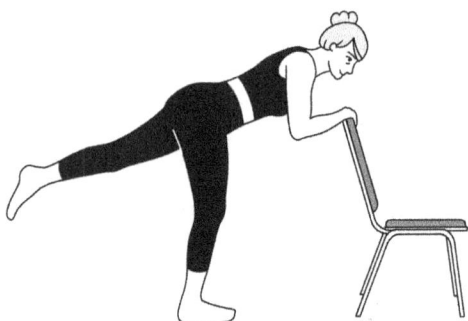

ASSISTED WARRIOR III POSE

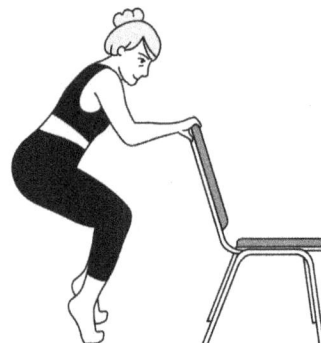

ASSISTED AWKWARD POSE

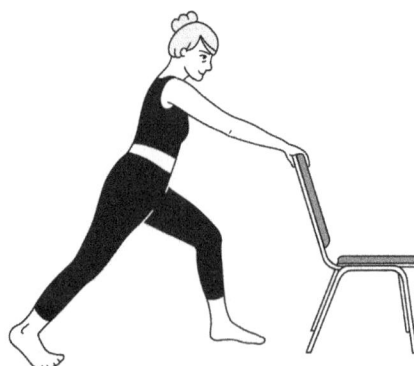

ASSISTED HIGH LUNGE POSE

Mountain Pose

- Stand with your back straight in front of a chair that is propped securely against a wall.

- Place your feet hip-distance apart, and press the soles of your feet into the ground. (Feel "all four corners" of your feet pressing firmly down).

- Relax your arms by your side with palms facing forward.

- Take a few breaths to ground yourself.

SUGGESTED MODIFICATIONS

To **decrease the challenge**, you can do this pose seated in the chair.

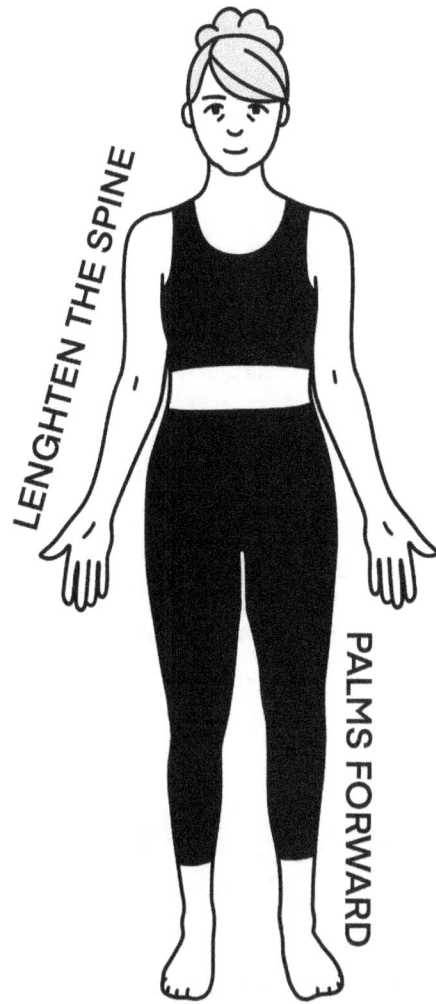

LENGHTEN THE SPINE

PALMS FORWARD

Assisted Chair Pose

- Place your hands on the back of the chair and exhale as you bend your knees.

- Lower your buttocks toward the floor, as if you want to sit in a chair. Keep your core engaged and your chest lifted.

- Keep your neck and spine in line with each other, and gaze softly forward.

- Rise into a standing position and then lower again into Chair Pose. Exhale as you bend your knees, and inhale as you straighten your knees and return to standing.

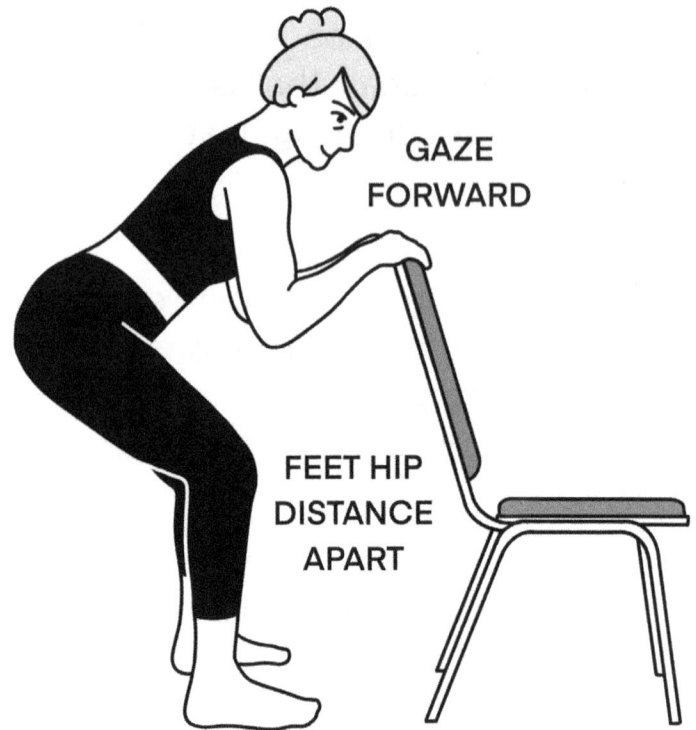

- Repeat 10-15 times.

GAZE FORWARD

FEET HIP DISTANCE APART

SUGGESTED MODIFICATIONS

To **increase the challenge**, hold onto the back of the chair with only one hand. To **decrease the challenge**, perform the Chair Pose sitting on the chair: your feet should still be hip-distance apart and pressing into the floor. Your arms will come up by your ears parallel to each other with the palms facing inwards. Lift your buttocks from the chair and hover just above the seat.

Assisted Warrior III Pose

- Stand tall and hold onto the back of the chair with both hands.

- Inhale to lengthen your spine, then exhale, transfer your weight to the right leg and begin to hinge forward.

- Keep your right leg as straight as you can without overstraining, then lift your left leg behind you.

- Keep your neck aligned with the rest of your spine.

- Engage your core and press into the right foot.

- Softly gaze forward.

- Rise into a standing position and then hinge forward again into Warrior III Pose. Exhale as you hinge forward, and inhale as you return to standing.

- Repeat 8-10 times on each side.

PRESS INTO THE ANCHORED FOOT

KEEP NECK ALIGNED

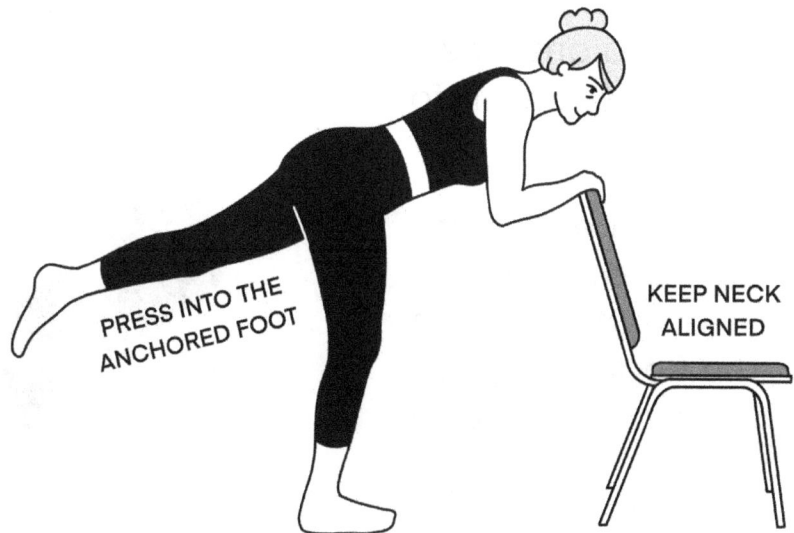

SUGGESTED MODIFICATIONS

To **increase the challenge**, hold onto the chair with only one hand. The other arm reaches forward toward the wall. To decrease the challenge, don't hinge as far forward.

Assisted Awkward Pose

- Stand tall with your feet hip-width apart, and hold onto the back of the chair for support.

- Exhale, bend your knees, and lower your buttocks toward the floor, as if you want to sit in a chair.

- Engage your core and lift your chest. Keep your neck and spine in line with each other, and gaze softly forward.

- From this crouched position, lift and lower your heels while keeping your knees bent. Inhale as you lift your heels and exhale as you lower your heels.

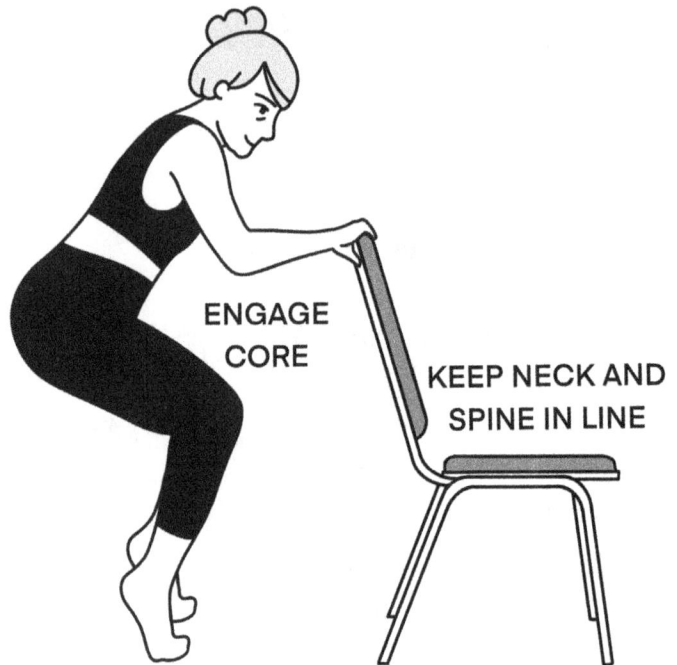

- Repeat 10-15 times.

ENGAGE CORE

KEEP NECK AND SPINE IN LINE

SUGGESTED MODIFICATIONS

To **increase the challenge**, you can hold onto the back of the chair with only one hand. To **decrease the challenge**, perform Awkward Pose while sitting on the chair: your feet should still be hip-distance apart and pressing into the floor. Your arms will come up by your ears parallel to each other with the palms facing inwards. Lift and lower your heels from this seated position.

Assisted High Lunge Pose

- Stand tall and hold onto the back of the chair. Exhale as you step your right foot back and stand on the ball of your right foot with your right heel lifted.

- Keep the right knee straight without locking it.

- Anchor the left foot into the ground and engage your left knee so that it doesn't fall in toward the midline.

- Gaze forward, lift your spine, and engage your core.

- Alternate between bending your front knee into High Lunge Pose on an exhale and straightening your front knee on an inhale.

- Repeat 8-10 times on each side.

TOES POINTING FORWARD

KEEP NECK ALIGNED

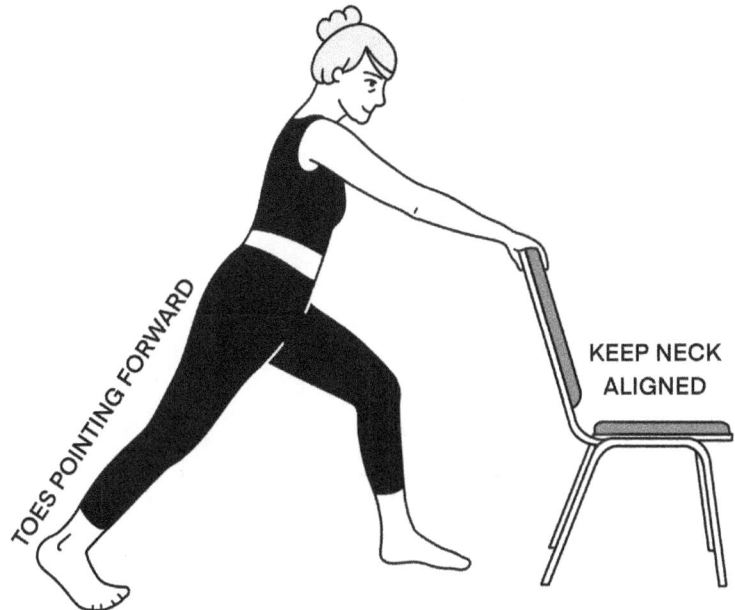

SUGGESTED MODIFICATIONS

To **increase the challenge**, release one hand from the chair and lift the arm straight overhead. To **decrease the challenge**, take a smaller step with the back leg so that you have more balance.

YOGA SEQUENCES FOR STRENGTH-BUILDING

SEQUENCE 2: YOGA FOR UPPER BODY STRENGTH

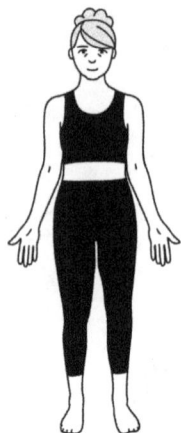

MOUNTAIN POSE

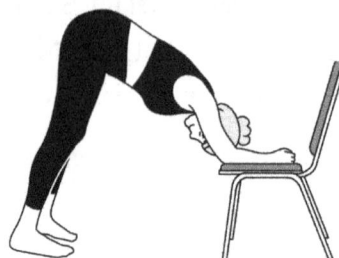

MODIFIED DOLPHIN POSE

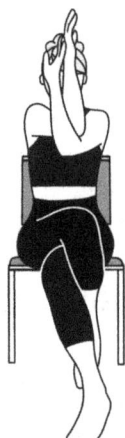

SEATED EAGLE POSE

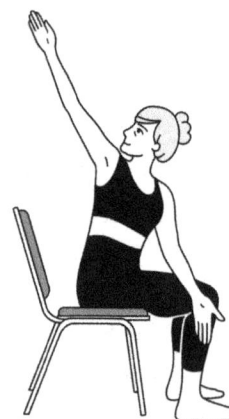

SEATED REVOLVED CHAIR POSE

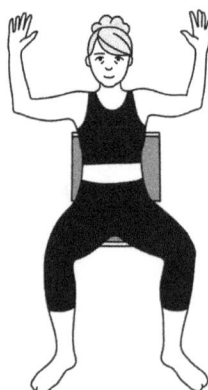

SEATED GODDESS POSE

Mountain Pose

- Prop your chair securely against a wall, then hold onto the back of the chair, place your feet hip-distance apart, and press the soles of your feet into the ground.

- Relax your arms by your side with palms facing forward.

- Take a few breaths to ground yourself.

SUGGESTED MODIFICATIONS

To **decrease the challenge**, you can do this pose seated in the chair.

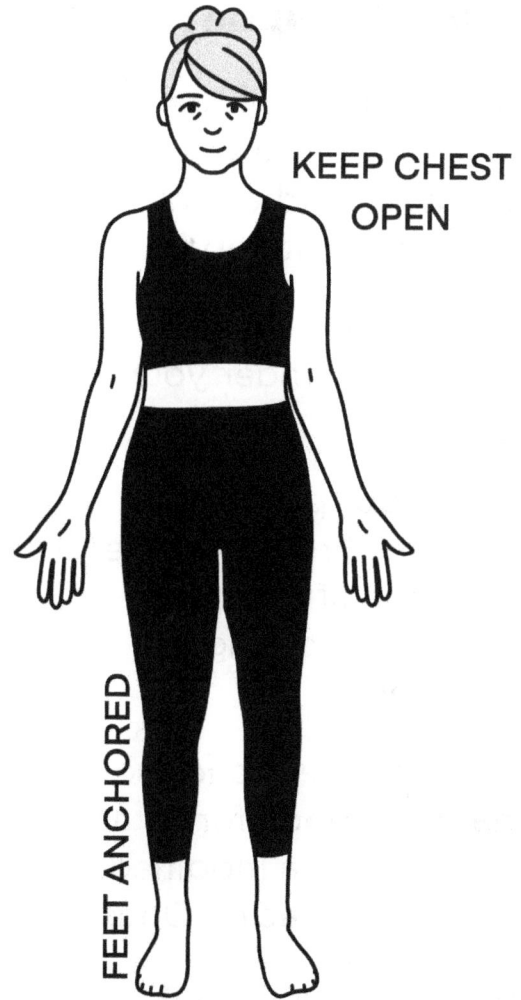

KEEP CHEST OPEN

FEET ANCHORED

Modified Dolphin Pose

- Kneel in front of the chair and place your forearms on the seat, shoulder-width apart.

- Your elbows should be directly under your shoulder.

- Press your palms and forearms firmly into the chair and lift your hips toward the ceiling on an exhale.

- Walk your feet back so that your body forms a 'V' shape or a modified Downward Facing Dog.

- Relax your neck and gaze towards your feet.

- Engage your core and press through your palms and forearms.

- Hold the pose for a few breaths, then release slowly and come back to kneeling.

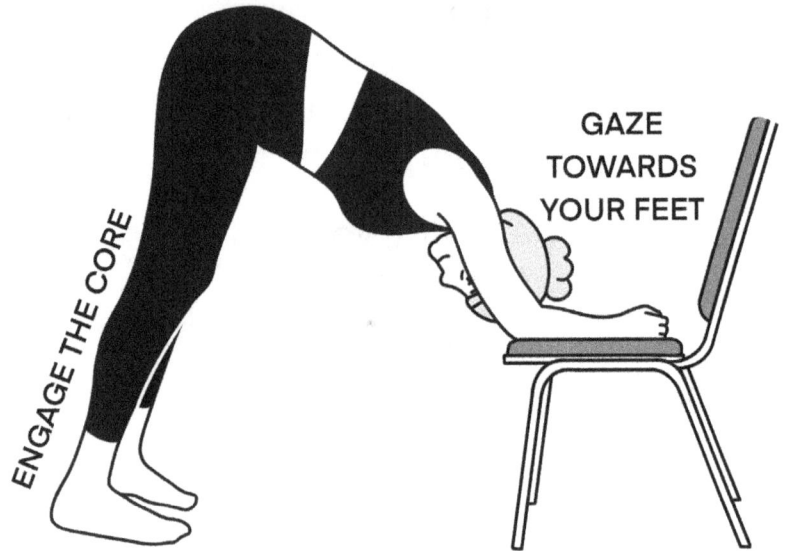

ENGAGE THE CORE

GAZE TOWARDS YOUR FEET

SUGGESTED MODIFICATIONS

To **increase the challenge**, step your feet further away from the chair. To **decrease the challenge**, you can remain in a kneeling position and focus on pressing your palms and forearms into the chair.

Seated Eagle Pose

- Take a seated position on the chair.

- Inhale as you lengthen your spine, then exhale and cross your right thigh over your left thigh and wrap your right foot around your left calf.

- Cross your right arm under your left arm and bend your elbows, trying to touch your palms together.

- Keep your elbows at shoulder height and imagine sliding forwards on your rib cage.

- Press your thighs and palms into each other as much as possible.

- Hold the pose for a few breaths, then release.

- Repeat on the other side.

HOLD THE POSE

KEEP HIPS ANCHORED

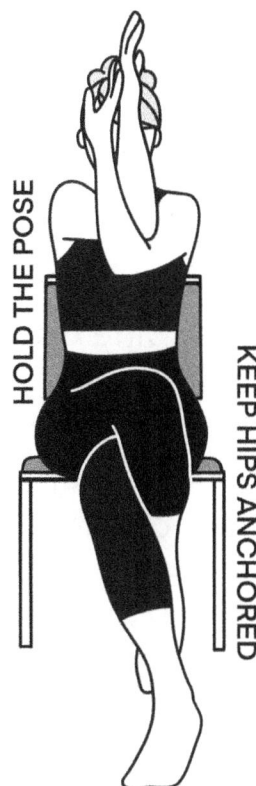

SUGGESTED MODIFICATIONS

To **increase the challenge**, you can take an assisted Eagle Pose in a standing position. Hold onto the chair with one or two hands and take Eagle legs (crossing one leg over the other). To **decrease the challenge**, cross your leg over your thigh without wrapping it around the calf. If you can't cross your arms in Eagle, wrap your arms around your chest to grab your shoulder blades on either side.

Seated Revolved Chair Pose

- Take a seated position with your feet together, and press through the bottoms of your feet.

- Lengthen your spine on an inhale, then exhale and twist your torso to the right, bringing your left hand to the outside of your right knee.

- Align your right arm and left arms, and point straight up toward the ceiling.

- Gaze straight ahead or toward your top hand, if it feels comfortable.

- Hold the twist for a few breaths while pressing your bottom arm into your knee.

- Release and repeat on the other side.

KEEP HIPS LEVEL

KEEP FEET ANCHORED

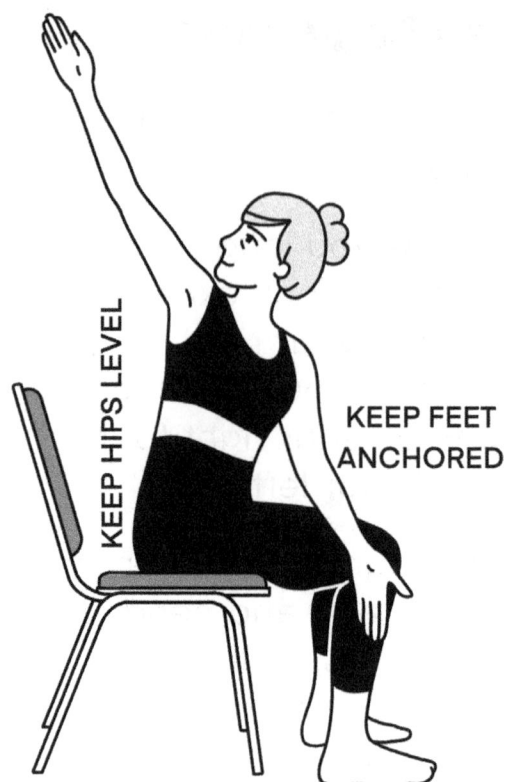

SUGGESTED MODIFICATIONS

To **increase the challenge**, do this pose while standing. The bottom hand will still be pressing into your knee and the top hand will be holding onto the back of the chair. To **decrease the challenge**, while performing Seated Revolved Chair Pose, do not twist as deep. Press the bottom hand into your knee, but keep your other hand on the back of the chair instead of lifting it toward the ceiling.

Seated Goddess Pose

- Take a seated position and lengthen through your spine.

- Exhale and place your feet wider than hip-distance apart with your toes pointing out.

- Lift your arms out to the sides so your elbows and shoulders are at a 90-degree angle, like a cactus.

- Spread your fingers wide and gently squeeze your shoulder blades together.

- Alternate between lifting your arms straight up and bringing them back into a cactus position to squeeze your shoulder blades.

- Inhale as you raise your arms and exhale as you cactus your arms. Repeat 10-15 times.

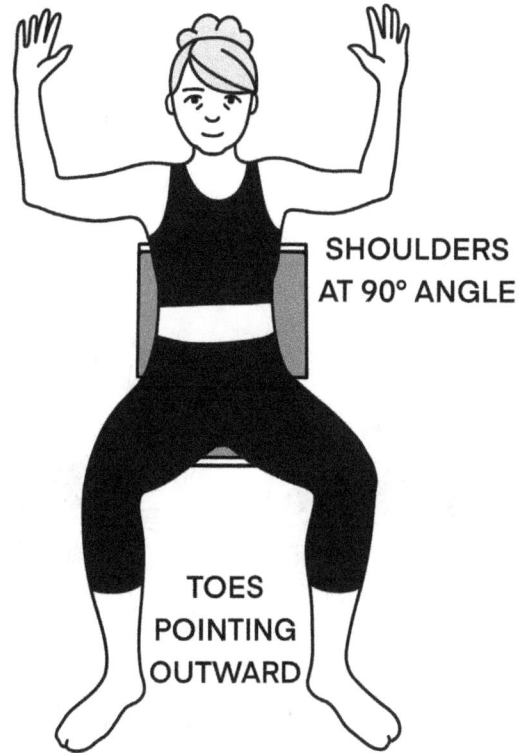

SHOULDERS AT 90° ANGLE

TOES POINTING OUTWARD

SUGGESTED MODIFICATIONS

To **decrease the challenge**, keep your hands together at the heart center. To **increase the challenge**, push through your feet and try to lift your buttocks from the chair.

YOGA SEQUENCES FOR STRENGTH-BUILDING

SEQUENCE 3: YOGA FOR CORE STRENGTH

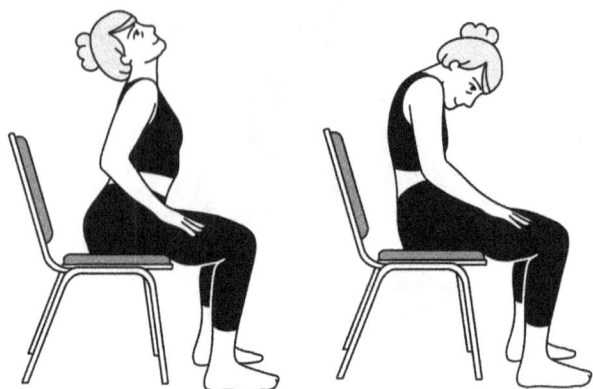

SEATED CAT AND COW POSE

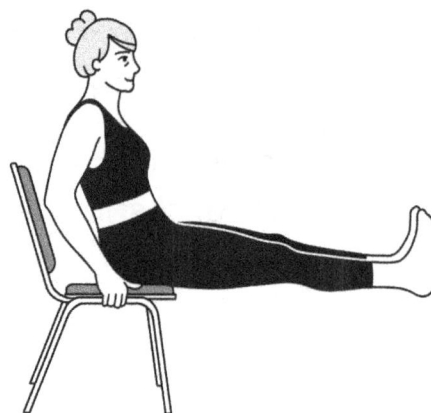

SEATED BOAT POSE

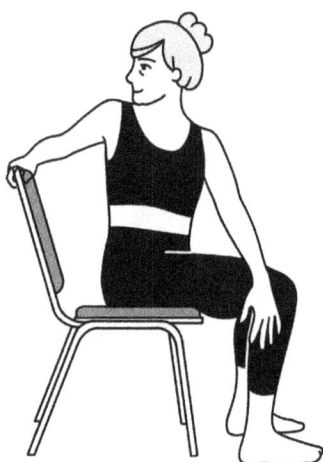

CHAIR SEATED TWIST

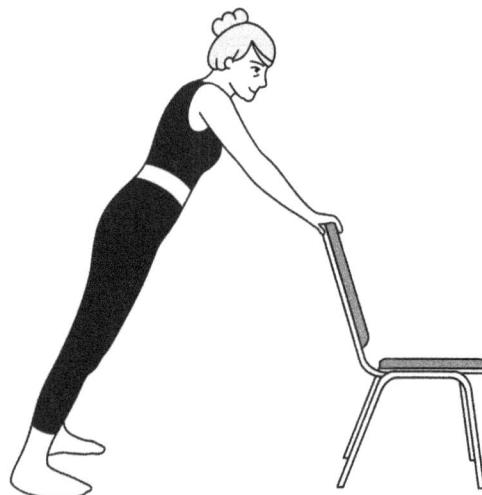

CHAIR PLANK POSE

Seated Cat and Cow Pose

- Sit in a chair that is propped up against a wall, lengthen your spine, and place your feet hip-distance apart.

- Rest both hands on your thighs.

- Inhale as you arch your back and lift your sternum toward the ceiling for Cow Pose.

- Engage your core and exhale as you round your back and bring your chin toward your chest for Cat Pose.

- Alternate between these two positions while syncing your movement to your breath.

- Repeat for a few breaths.

ARCH INWARD

FEET ANCHORED

STRETCH THE LOWER BACK

ARCH OUTWARD

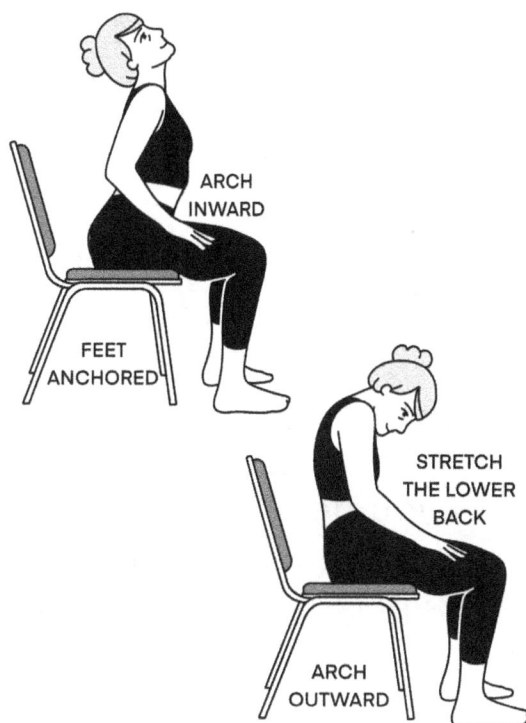

Seated Boat Pose

- Take a seated position and lengthen through the spine.

- Exhale as you lean back slightly while holding onto the sides of the seat.

- Engage your core and lift your feet off the ground with your knees straight.

- Lift your chest, straighten your spine, and hold the pose for a few breaths.

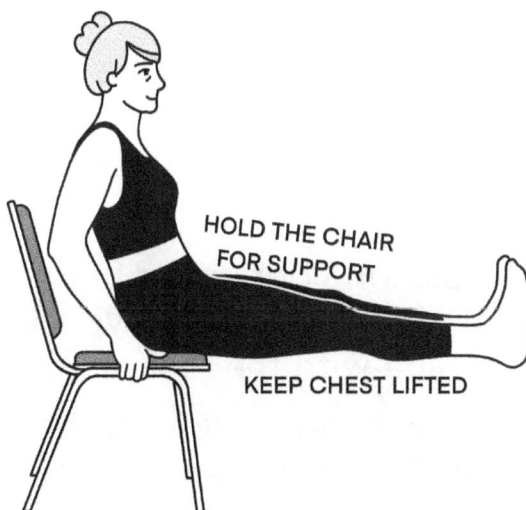

HOLD THE CHAIR FOR SUPPORT

KEEP CHEST LIFTED

SUGGESTED MODIFICATIONS

To **increase the challenge**, lean further back into the position. To **decrease the challenge**, keep your knees bent instead of having them straight.

Chair Seated Twist

- Sit tall, inhale as you lengthen your spine, and exhale as you twist to the right.

- Hold onto the back of the chair with your right hand, and press your left hand into your right thigh.

- Inhale to lengthen your spine, engage your core and exhale as you deepen the twist.

- Lift your chest, relax your shoulders, and hold the pose for a few breaths.

- Release and repeat on the other side.

KEEP CHEST UP

SHOULDERS RELAXED

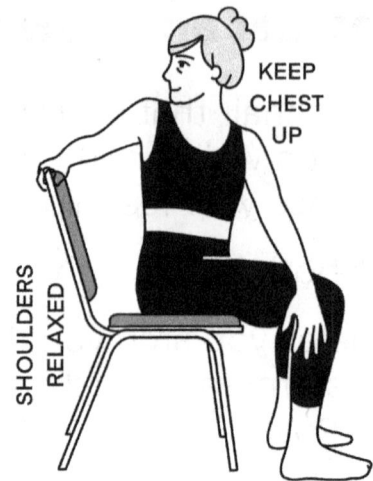

SUGGESTED MODIFICATIONS

To **decrease the challenge**, do not go as deep into your twist.

Chair Plank Pose

- Stand in front of the chair and place your hands on the seat.

- Exhale as you extend your legs back into a modified plank position.

- Keep your elbows and knees straight, but not locked.

- Position your wrists under your shoulders and keep your neck in line with the rest of your spine.

- Engage your core and hold the position for a few breaths.

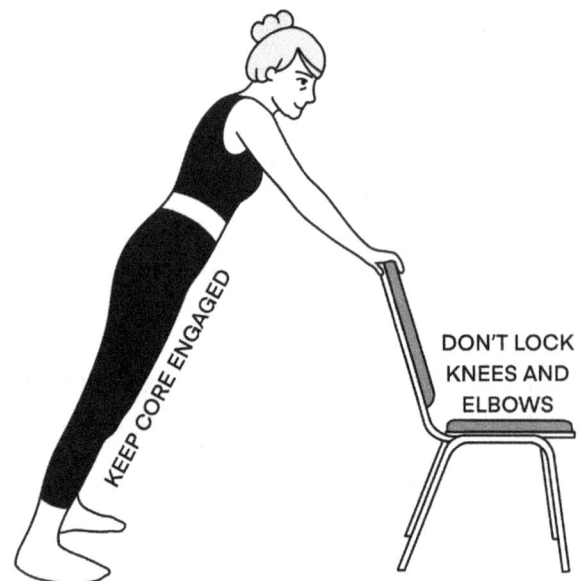

KEEP CORE ENGAGED

DON'T LOCK KNEES AND ELBOWS

SUGGESTED MODIFICATIONS

To **increase the challenge**, pull one knee towards your chest at a time, as if you're climbing a mountain. Exhale as you bring your knee toward your chest and inhale as you extend the leg out. To **decrease the challenge**, reduce the distance you step your feet back, so your body is on less of an incline.

YOGA SEQUENCES FOR STRENGTH-BUILDING

SEQUENCE 4: YOGA FOR FULL BODY STRENGTH

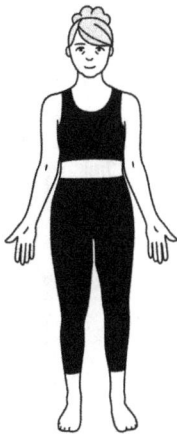

MOUNTAIN POSE

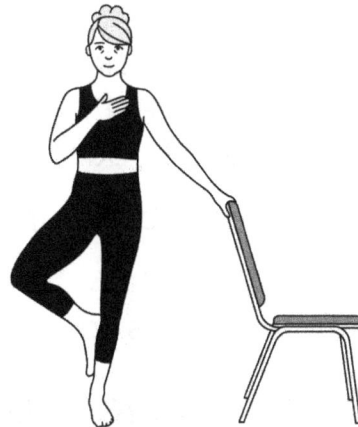

ASSISTED TREE POSE

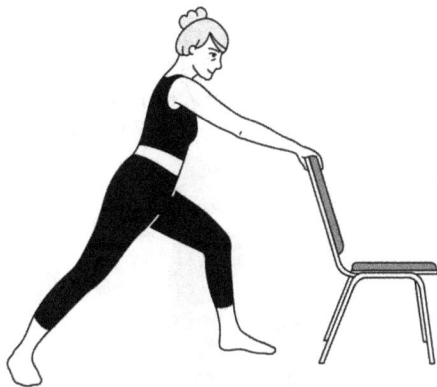

ASSISTED WARRIOR I POSE

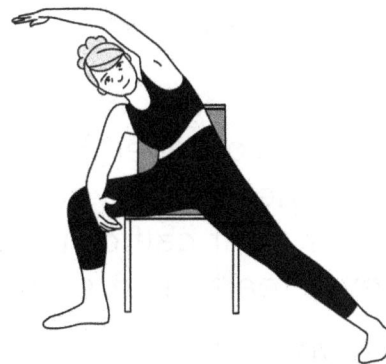

SIDE ANGLE POSE

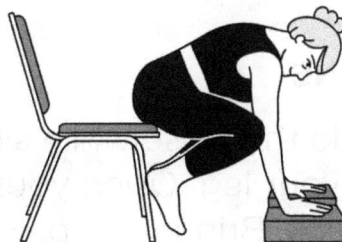

SEATED CROW POSE

Mountain Pose

- Prop your chair securely against the wall.

- Stand with your back straight in front of the chair, place your feet hip-distance apart, and press the soles of your feet into the ground.

- Relax your arms by your side with palms facing forward.

- Take a few breaths to ground yourself.

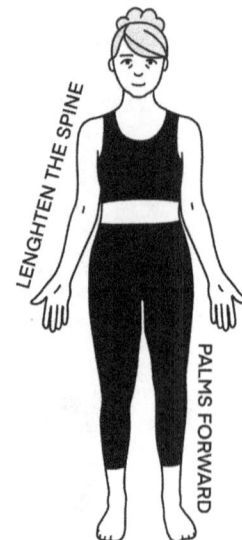

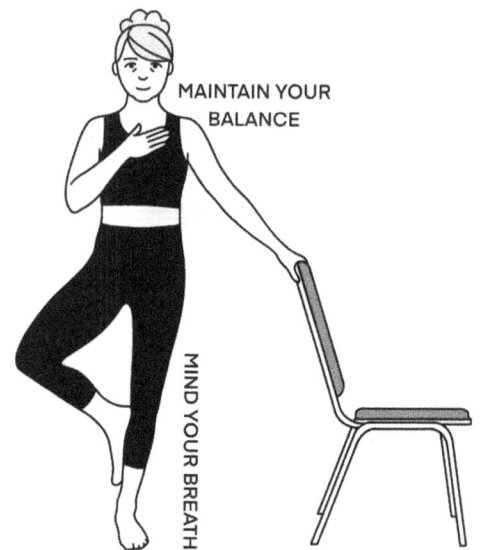

SUGGESTED MODIFICATIONS

To **decrease the challenge**, you can do this pose seated in the chair.

LENGHTEN THE SPINE

PALMS FORWARD

Assisted Tree Pose

- Hold onto the back of the chair, inhale as you shift your weight onto your right foot, and then place your left foot on your inner right calf or inner right thigh, whichever feels most comfortable.

- Engage your core and lengthen through your spine.

- Focus your gaze straight forward, and hold the pose for a few breaths as you try to maintain your balance on the right leg.

- Release your leg and repeat on the opposite side.

MAINTAIN YOUR BALANCE

MIND YOUR BREATH

SUGGESTED MODIFICATIONS

To **decrease the challenge**, do this pose while sitting on the chair. Press one foot into the floor to anchor your leg. Open your other leg out to the side as you rest your foot on a block. Bring your palms together at your heart. To **increase the challenge**, in the standing Tree Pose, hold onto the back of the chair with only one hand and place the other hand at your heart center.

Assisted Warrior I Pose

- Hold onto the chair, place your feet hip-distance apart, inhale to lengthen your spine, then exhale and step your right foot back into a lunge.

- Keep your left knee bent and your right leg straight.

- Turn the foot of the back leg out to a 45-degree angle.

- Hold the pose and breathe.

- On an inhale, extend your front knee, and on the exhale, bend your front knee back into Warrior I Pose.

- Repeat 8-10 times on each side while connecting your movement to your breath.

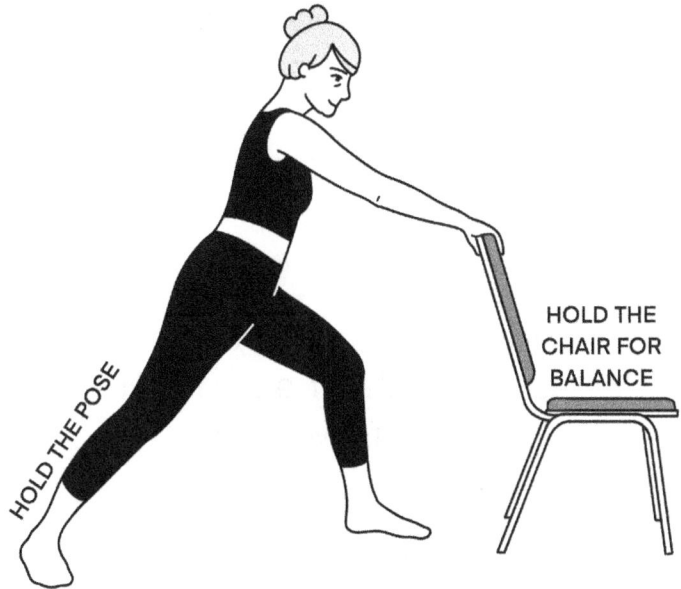

HOLD THE POSE

HOLD THE CHAIR FOR BALANCE

SUGGESTED MODIFICATIONS

To **increase the challenge**, hold onto the chair with only one hand. Raise your other arm overhead with the palm facing inward. To **decrease the challenge**, take a smaller step backward so that it is easier to balance.

Side Angle Pose

- Sit tall, inhale as you lengthen your spine, and exhale as you open your right knee out to the side and point your toes to the right. Keep your right knee bent at about 90 degrees.

- Extend your left leg back so it forms a straight line and point your left toes forward.

- Rest your right forearm against your right thigh and extend your left arm overhead.

- Create a straight line from your left foot to your right fingertips.

- You can look up toward the ceiling, or straight ahead, whichever feels gentler on your neck.

- To increase the demand on your core, keep your leg position the same, and then exhale as you lean into a side angle position, and inhale as you lift and straighten your torso. Repeat 8-10 times.

- Repeat the same exercise on the opposite side.

FEEL THE STRETCH

POINT TOES FORWARD

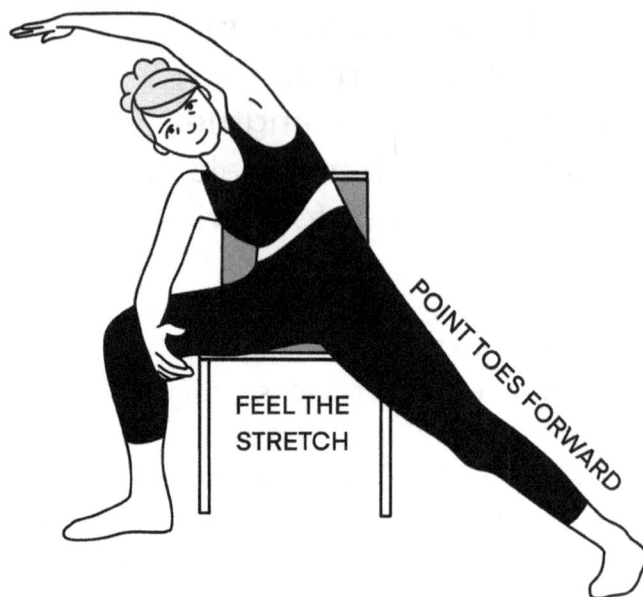

SUGGESTED MODIFICATIONS

To **decrease the challenge**, hold the extended side angle position for 8-10 breaths on each side instead of alternating between sitting upright and bending into the extended position.

Seated Crow Pose

- Place two yoga blocks on the floor in front of you.

- Sit tall with your buttocks close to the edge of the chair and your feet at hip distance apart.

- Exhale as you lean forward and bring your hands to the blocks.

- Your forearms should be between your legs and pressing against your inner knees.

- Bend your knees to lift your feet off the ground and bring them back under the chair, keep your feet pointing down.

- Press into the blocks to keep your body stable.

- Stay here for a few breaths before coming back to a seated position.

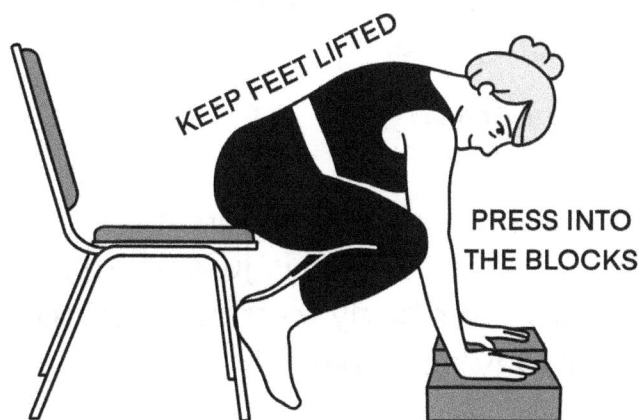

KEEP FEET LIFTED

PRESS INTO THE BLOCKS

SUGGESTED MODIFICATIONS

To **increase the challenge**, press harder into the blocks and try to imagine you want to lift your seat off from the chair. To **decrease the challenge**, bring the blocks to a taller height or keep your hands pressing onto your thighs.

COOL DOWN AND MEDITATION

8

"Almost everything will work again if you unplug it for a few minutes, including you."

Anne Lamott

We discussed the importance of warming up the body before physical activity; it is just as important to cool down. A cool down allows your body to transition from physical activity back to your everyday activities.

The benefits include **returning heart rate back to baseline** (especially for more strenuous cardio or strength yoga sequences), **enhancing recovery** (it brings us back to a state of rest so our body can recuperate), and **improving psychological health** (it allows you to feel the mental benefits of exercise, like an improved mood and a sense of well-being and gratitude).

The best part of cooling down is that it doesn't have to be lengthy to be beneficial. Taking five minutes at the end of an exercise session can be enough to lower your heart rate back to baseline.

The cool down routine that follows is one you can always come back to at the end of your chair yoga session. It also works well as well as a meditation practice for your mental and emotional health.

COOL DOWN AND RELAXATION SERIES

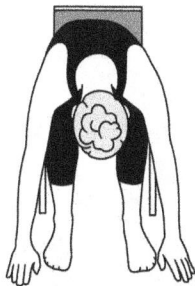

SEATED FORWARD FOLD

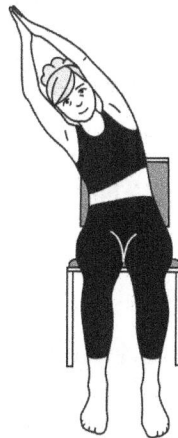

SEATED SIDE BEND POSE

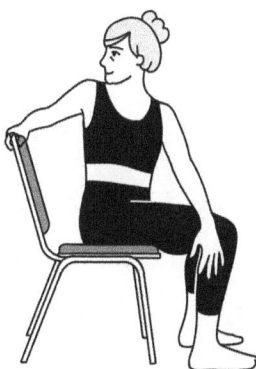

CHAIR SEATED TWIST

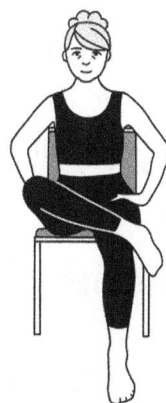

SEATED PIGEON POSE

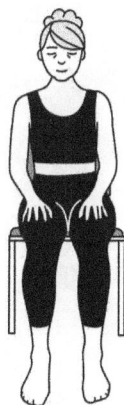

SEATED SAVASANA

Seated Forward Fold

- Prop your chair up against a wall, if you haven't done so already.

- Begin in a tall seated position, and place your feet hip distance apart.

- Inhale to lengthen your spine, and exhale while folding forward.

- Rest your fingertips on the ground, or on your thighs, whichever is more comfortable.

- Relax your shoulders, and let your head be heavy.

- Hold the pose for a few breaths before rising back to a sitting position with an inhale.

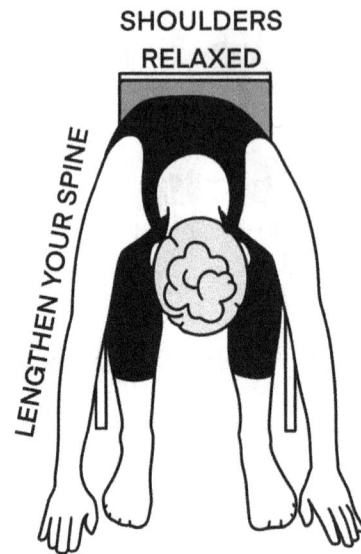

Seated Side Bend Pose

- Sit with your spine tall, and lift your arms overhead on an inhale.

- Interlace your fingers leaving out your thumb and index on each hand.

- Exhale and extend to the right.

- Press both feet into the ground.

- Hold for a few breaths and feel the stretch in the left side body.

- Inhale as you bring your arms back to center, exhale to release your arms by your side.

- Repeat on the left side.

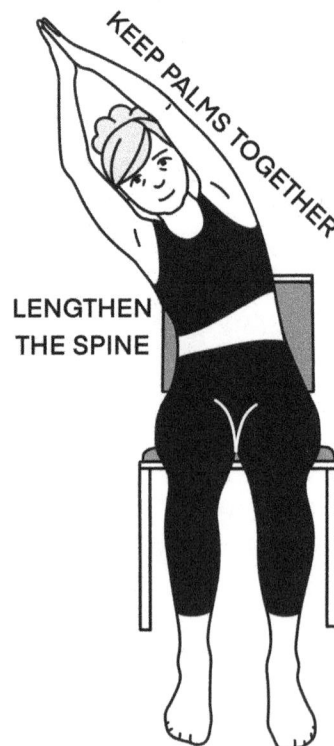

Chair Seated Twist

- Inhale to lengthen your spine, then exhale as you twist to the right.

- Hold onto the back of the chair with your right hand, and press your left hand into your right thigh.

- Inhale to lengthen your spine, and exhale to twist further into the movement by engaging your core.

- Lift your chest and relax your shoulders as you deepen the twist.

- Hold the pose for a few breaths, then repeat on the left side.

- Inhale and return to center.

KEEP CHEST UP

SHOULDERS RELAXED

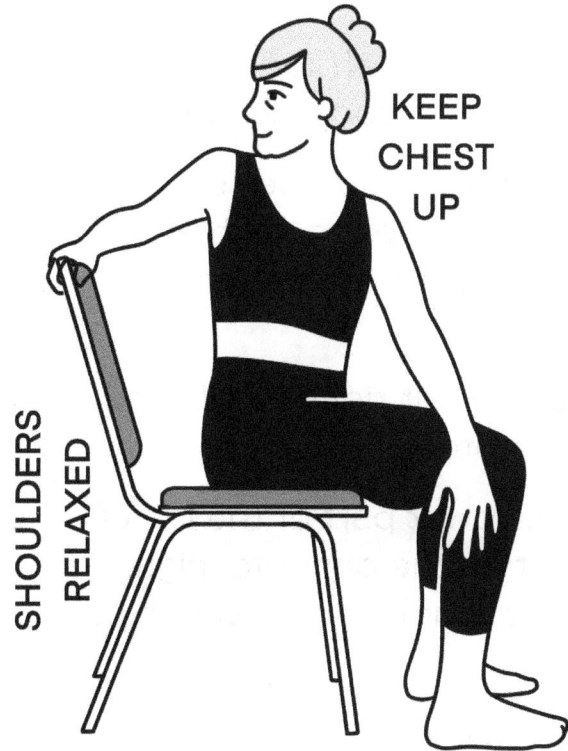

SUGGESTED MODIFICATIONS

To **decrease the challenge**, do not twist as far when you rotate your torso.

Seated Pigeon Pose

- Press your left foot into the floor to anchor the leg.

- Bring the right foot up and press it into the anchored leg to create the shape of a number 4.

- Keep your right foot flexed to protect your knee.

- The lower part of the leg can rest on the opposite thigh. Rest your hands on your hips.

- Engage your core, lengthen your spine, and focus your gaze straight forward.

- Hold the pose for a few breaths. Then repeat on the left leg.

- Exhale as you release both legs and anchor both feet on the floor.

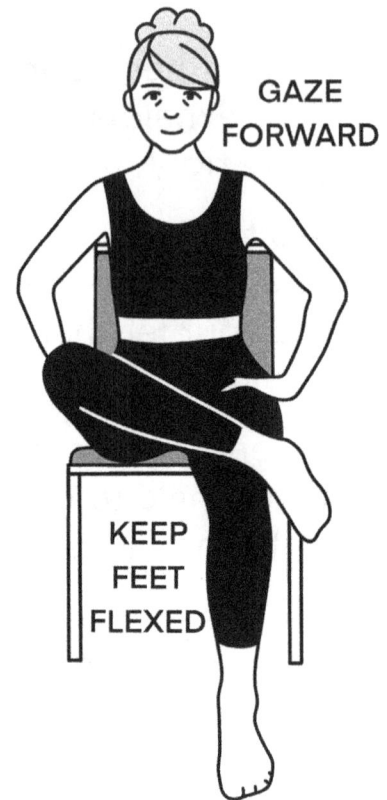

GAZE FORWARD

KEEP FEET FLEXED

SUGGESTED MODIFICATIONS

To **increase the challenge**, press gently on the bent knee to increase the stretch in your hip, or lean your torso forward.

Seated Savasana

- Keep your feet hip-distance apart, your spine tall, and your shoulders relaxed.

- Rest your hands on your thighs, turn your focus inward, and close your eyes.

- Breathe naturally, try to stay present, and enjoy the moment of relaxation.

- If your mind wanders, gently bring your attention back to your breath.

- Stay in Savasana for as long as you like, but aim for at least two minutes.

- When you are ready to end your practice, gently open your eyes, and try to move mindfully into the next steps of your day.

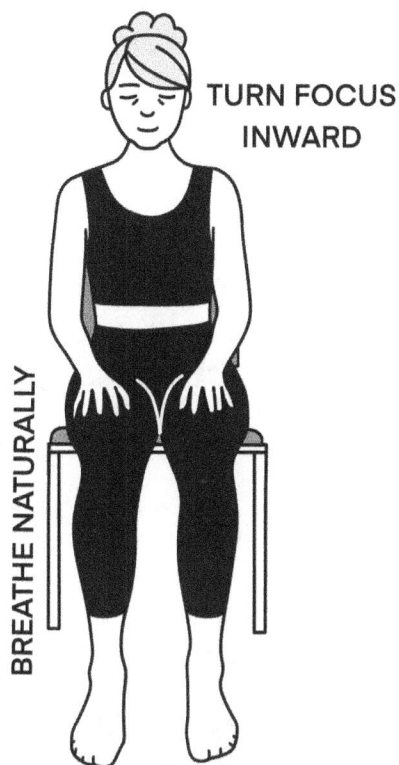

TURN FOCUS INWARD

BREATHE NATURALLY

SUGGESTED MODIFICATIONS

To increase comfort, use a cushion to support your lower back against the seat of the chair. If you feel uncomfortable with your eyes closed, keep them open and gaze softly forward.

MEDITATION ENHANCES WELL-BEING

Meditation can promote mental and emotional well-being. According to the National Center for Complementary and Integrative Health (NCCIH), meditation includes a range of techniques that aim to integrate the mind and body, promoting mental calmness and improving overall well-being. There are different types of meditation which range from focusing on the breath, a sound, or a specific sensation; visualization; or repeating certain words or phrases, called mantras.

Mindfulness is a type of meditation that entails maintaining attention on the present without any judgment. Below we will present to you a mindfulness meditation practice that you can come back to daily. This can be a stand-alone practice or as part of your cool down

MINDFULNESS MEDITATION PRACTICE:

- Sit comfortably on a chair in an area free of distractions. Relax your shoulders and take three full breaths.

- Close your eyes and turn your focus inward, and begin mentally scanning your body, from your head and down to your toes. Notice areas of comfort and discomfort. There is no need to change anything: simply observe.

- Then, start again at the top with your head, draw your attention to each muscle, and this time try to release the tension.

- On an inhale, slowly move your attention down your body to the next muscle, and on an exhale, imagine the tension is melting away.

- After releasing all the tension, from your head to your toes, take a moment to observe the change in your state of relaxation.

- Now, bring your attention to your breath and notice how your rib cage expands as you inhale and relaxes as you exhale. Imagine the air entering your lungs and leaving your lungs, releasing any remaining tension in your body.

- Stay here for about 10 breaths.

- Try to stay present during this meditation practice. Every time you feel your mind wandering, bring your attention back to the breath. Whenever you lose focus, simply return your attention to your breath.

- When you feel ready, bring your attention back to your surroundings, and feel your body pressing against the chair, and slowly open your eyes.

WEIGHT LOSS MANAGEMENT

"Let go of the things that no longer serve you, and put your problems in the past where they belong." Lisa Lieberman-Wang

The research on yoga for weight loss in older adults remains limited; more quality research is needed for this specific subset of the population. However, **regular yoga practice has been shown to help with weight management** in other populations, specifically in overweight and obese individuals as well as women in their 30s to 50s.

A study by Lauche et al. (2016), published in Preventative Medicine, found that yoga was a safe and effective method to decrease Body Mass Index (BMI) in overweight and obese individuals. Another study took 60 women and separated them into two groups. One group did yoga twice per week and the other took cooking and nutrition classes. Both groups had previously done three months of behavioral treatment for weight loss.

They found that both groups had similar results in weight loss. However, what was interesting was that the women who initially lost more than 5% of body fat from the behavioral treatment, had better long-term weight loss if they were in the yoga group. The women in the yoga group also had better tolerance to stress, more mindfulness, and more self-compassion (Unick et al., 2022). Yoga benefits people who are overweight, and may help with long-term weight loss for people of all ages.

A BALANCED DIET IS ESSENTIAL FOR WEIGHT LOSS

You cannot lose weight if you only do a few yoga sequences per week; weight management is more successful when used along with other powerful tools, like walking and a balanced diet. What exactly does a balanced diet look like?

As a general guideline, the Center for Disease Control (CDC) recommends that adults **focus on fruits, vegetables, whole grains, and fat-free or low-fat dairy**. Additionally, it is important to incorporate foods with protein like seafood, lean meat, poultry, eggs, legumes, soy products, nuts, and seeds. A healthy diet should also be low in sugar, salt, saturated fats, trans fats, and cholesterol.

Finally, try to **remain within your individual calorie needs**. Generally, adult women need 2,000 calories per day and adult men need 2,500 calories per day. However, your daily calorie intake can also vary depending on your level of physical activity, and whether or not you are actively trying to lose weight.

A good resource to determine your daily calorie intake is to use the MyPlate Plan calculator available at https://www.myplate.gov/myplate-plan. It will determine how many calories you need based on your age, sex, weight, height, and physical activity level. However, if you need a more personalized approach to nutrition because of specific dietary requirements or specific weight goals, it's always better to consult with a registered dietician.

WALKING DAILY SUPPORTS WEIGHT LOSS

Evidence shows that walking 30 minutes five times per week can help reduce body weight and body fat when used in combination with a diet plan (Bond et al., 2002).

A meta-analysis published in the Annals of Family Medicine found that walking with a pedometer-based approach, without the use of a diet plan, also contributed to a small weight loss of 0.05 kg per week. The participants across different studies walked on average 2,000 to 4,000 steps or more per day, and the longer they walked, the more weight they lost (Richardson et al., 2008).

Walking can be a powerful tool to help with weight loss, and it becomes even more useful when combined with a healthy diet plan. Try to walk 30 minutes per day most days of the week; it will lead to improved health and help in achieving weight goals.

To sum up, to manage weight, focus on maintaining a healthy and balanced diet, and incorporate regular physical activity, such as yoga and walking most days of the week.

In the next chapter, we will present to you the 28-day challenge which will include a daily plan of yoga sequences for different ability and fitness levels.

"The most difficult thing is the decision to act, the rest is merely tenacity."

Amelia Earhart

By this point, you have learned all the chair yoga sequences presented in the previous chapters. Now, it's time to integrate this learning into a 28-day plan. Below are some tables with the suggested yoga sequences for each week. Please refer to the instructions provided to perform each yoga pose safely and correctly.

Each week, you will perform five mini-workouts or five combinations of sequences. You will notice that there are two rest days per week from yoga included in the tables. Feel free to take more rest days as needed and always listen to your body first. Each day includes a warm-up, a workout (yoga sequence), and a cool-down. Each week is designed to increase the challenge; however, look at the suggested modifications for poses if you need to make them easier.

In addition to the chair yoga sequences, we also recommend that you **walk for 30 minutes, at least five times per week**. Adjust the suggested walking routine to suit your personal needs. For instance, you can divide your walking into separate sessions and walk three times a day for 10 minutes, or two times a day for 15 minutes. Every little bit of movement counts! The most important thing is to prioritize your safety and stay within your limits.

WEEKLY GOALS

Remember to stay consistent and let your body adjust. As you progress, you should notice subtle improvements to your sense of mindfulness and flow.

WEEK 1: Learn the new movements, and link breath to movement as you practice.

WEEK 2: Begin building strength and balance.

WEEK 3: Integrate cardio exercise.

WEEK 4: Focus on mindfulness and meditation.

WEEK 1

Goal: Learn the new movements, and link breath to movement as you practice.

	WARM UP	WORK OUT	COOL DOWN
MONDAY	Seated shoulder rolls; Seated neck rolls; Seated marches	Sequence 3: Chair slow flow	Seated savasana
TUESDAY	Seated ankle and wrist rotation; Seated cat and cow pose; Seated marches	Sequence 1: Balance and hip opener	Chair seated twist; Seated savasana
WEDNESDAY	Seated cat and cow pose; Seated side bend pose; Chair seated twist	Seated moon salutation series	Seated forward fold; Seated savasana
THURSDAY	Rest	Rest	Rest
FRIDAY	Seated ankle and wrist rotation; Seated cat and cow pose; Seated marches	Sequence 1: Balance and hip opener	Chair seated twist; Seated savasana
SATURDAY	Seated shoulder rolls; Seated neck rolls; Seated cat and cow pose	Seated sun salutation series	Chair seated twist, Seated pigeon pose; Seated savasana
SUNDAY	Rest	Rest	Rest

WEEK 2

Goal: Begin building strength and balance.

	WARM UP	WORK OUT	COOL DOWN
MONDAY	Seated ankle and wrist rotation; Seated shoulder rolls; Seated side bend pose	Sequence 2: Posterior flexibility and balance	Seated pigeon pose; Chair seated twist, Seated savasana
TUESDAY	Chair seated twist, Seated cat and cow pose; Seated ankle and wrist rotation; Seated shoulder rolls	Sequence 2: Yoga for upper body strength	Mindfulness & meditation practice
WEDNESDAY	Seated neck rolls; Seated shoulder rolls; Seated ankle and wrist rotation; Chair seated twist	Sequence 4: Backbend and balance	Seated forward fold; Seated pigeon pose; Seated savasana
THURSDAY	Rest	Rest	Rest
FRIDAY	Seated cat and cow pose; Seated ankle and wrist rotation; Seated marches	Sequence 1: Yoga for lower body strength	Chair seated twist; Seated side bend pose; Seated savasana
SATURDAY	Seated shoulder rolls; Seated ankle and wrist rotation; Seated marches	Sequence 3: Back opener and balance	Chair seated twist; Seated side bend pose; Seated savasana
SUNDAY	Rest	Rest	Rest

WEEK 3

Goal: Integrate cardio exercise.

	WARM UP	WORK OUT	COOL DOWN
MONDAY	Seated shoulder rolls; Seated neck rolls; Seated side bend pose	Sequence 1: Chair warrior flow	Seated pigeon pose; Chair seated twist; Seated savasana
TUESDAY	Seated ankle and wrist rotation; Seated side bend pose; Seated marches	Sequence 3: Yoga for core strength	Mindfulness & meditation practice
WEDNESDAY	Seated ankle and wrist rotation; Seated shoulder rolls, Seated cat and cow pose; Seated marches	Sequence 2: Chair power flow	Seated forward fold; Chair seated twist; Seated savasana
THURSDAY	Rest	Rest	Rest
FRIDAY	Seated ankle and wrist rotation; Seated cat and cow pose; Seated side bend pose; Seated marches	Sequence 4: Yoga for full body strength	Chair seated twist; Seated pigeon pose; Seated savasana
SATURDAY	Seated shoulder rolls, Seated neck rolls; Seated cat and cow pose	Sequence 1: Chair warrior flow; Sequence 2: Chair power flow	Chair seated twist, Seated pigeon pose; Seated savasana
SUNDAY	Rest	Rest	Rest

WEEK 4

Goal: Focus on mindfulness and meditation.

	WARM UP	WORK OUT	COOL DOWN
MONDAY	Seated shoulder rolls, Seated neck rolls; Seated marches	Sequence 4: Backbend and balance; Sequence 2: Yoga for upper body strength	Chair seated twist; Seated savasana
TUESDAY	Seated ankle and wrist rotation; Seated shoulder rolls; Seated marches	Sequence 3: Back opener and balance; Sequence 2: Chair power flow	Chair seated twist, Seated pigeon pose; Seated savasana
WEDNESDAY	Seated cat and cow pose; Seated side bend pose; Chair seated twist	Sequence 1: Yoga for lower body strength; Sequence 3: Chair slow flow	Seated forward fold, Mindfulness & meditation practice
THURSDAY	Rest	Rest	Rest
FRIDAY	Seated ankle and wrist rotation; Seated cat and cow pose; Seated marches	Sequence 2: Posterior flexibility and balance; Sequence 3: Yoga for core strength	Seated forward fold, Mindfulness & meditation practice
SATURDAY	Seated sun salutation series	Sequence 4: Yoga for full body strength	Chair seated twist, Seated pigeon pose; Seated savasana
SUNDAY	Rest	Rest	Rest

BEYOND CHAIR YOGA

11

"As long as you keep going, you'll keep getting better. And as you get better, you gain more confidence. That alone is success."

Tamara Taylor

SUGGESTIONS FOR CONTINUING THE PRACTICE BEYOND THE 28-DAY CHALLENGE

Yoga is referred to as a practice, because there is always room for improvement and growth. After the 28-day challenge, your journey with yoga doesn't have to end. Below are some suggestions to keep you motivated to practice yoga beyond the 28-day challenge.

1. SET NEW GOALS

As you keep practicing yoga, it's a good idea to keep adjusting and modifying your goals. Having something to strive towards will keep you motivated and accountable.

Your next goal might focus on improving flexibility, balance, mobility, strength, or stamina. Or you might choose a goal that focuses on mindfulness or stress.

2. EXPAND YOUR YOGA PRACTICE

When your practice begins to feel easy, challenge yourself to try the more difficult variations, or increase your practice time, or practice more often. You could also look into going to in-person classes or taking up online classes to add some variety to your yoga practice. This will make you discover new poses and ways to practice as well as meet like-minded individuals.

TIPS FOR INTEGRATING YOGA INTO DAILY LIFE

Aim to integrate movement into your everyday routine. Here are a few tips on how to do so:

1. BREAK UP YOUR PRACTICE

If you're struggling to fit longer yoga sessions into your day, try breaking up your practice into shorter sessions. You could even select two or three poses from a yoga sequence to focus instead of an entire workout for mini sessions. Or, try to integrate a sequence at the same time every day in your morning routine or include it in your nighttime wind-down routine.

2. PRACTICE BREATHING AND MINDFULNESS THROUGHOUT THE DAY

Yoga is more than just physical exercise; it's also about practicing breathing and mindfulness, which can be integrated into moments throughout your day. For example, you can practice mindfulness when you're on a walk or accomplishing a quiet task. The goal is simply to be in the present moment and to focus your attention inward. When you find your mind wandering and racing throughout the day, this is the perfect time to put your mindfulness practice to good use.

You can also practice your breathing techniques throughout the day even if it's just for 5-10 breaths. You can do this at any time to help you find a more relaxed mode.

3. WORKPLACE INTEGRATION

If you work and your work requires sitting in a chair for long periods, you can easily integrate yoga into your work routine. Do one yoga pose every hour, focus on your breath for a 2-minute mindfulness practice every couple of hours. It can be helpful to set a timer to remind you to stretch and take some deep breaths. You decide how it could benefit you and how you want to fit it into your workday.

CONTINUING ON YOUR WEIGHT LOSS JOURNEY

Your weight loss journey goes beyond the 28-day challenge. There will be a point where you reach your goal weight, but the good habits you implement need to continue for a lifetime. It's easy to revert to old habits, so here are some tips to keep you on track:

1. STAY CONSISTENT

Consistency is essential when it comes to weight loss. This means on most days, it's important to keep up with some form of exercise or movement as well as having a balanced diet. To hold you accountable and help with consistency, it's a good idea to keep a log where you can write down your daily food intake and exercise which can include walking and yoga.

2. STAY ACTIVE

Be active most days of the week, whenever possible.

Movement or activity doesn't have to be in the same form all the time. Some people might find it more motivating to have a variety of ways to move their bodies. Walking is strongly encouraged on most days of the week. Then, you can add another form of activity such as yoga. On some days, you could also do swimming, biking, or even aerobic group classes to mix things up. The goal is to keep moving!

3. SEEK NUTRITIONAL GUIDANCE

If you have been trying to lose weight for a while and feel like you can't do so on your own, it might be time to seek some guidance from a professional. Dieticians can help to build you a nutritional plan and help you achieve your weight-loss goals.

CONCLUSION: KEEP GOING!

Staying motivated to keep practicing yoga is the most difficult part. Here are some tips for how to maintain a yoga practice.

1. KEEP A JOURNAL

It was previously mentioned that keeping a log of your food and exercise can help with consistency. In your journal, you can also write down your goals and your improvements or achievements. You can also write down what challenges you're experiencing. If you regularly check in and reflect on your progress, it can help you see how far you have come and stay on track.

2. JOIN A COMMUNITY

Another great way to stay motivated is to join a yoga community. This could be an online community, or an in-person yoga class. If possible, consider having tea after a yoga class with some of the other yogis, as a way to deepen the connection. Or join a yoga challenge to keep things fresh and interesting. Joining a community, no matter the format, is a great way to stay motivated and interact with like-minded people.

3. FIND YOUR INSPIRATION

Actively seek out motivation for your practice on a regular basis. There are many books on yoga and meditation that can inspire your practice, and in-person conferences or daylong workshops can be fun and energizing. With the internet at the tip of our fingers, it's now easier than ever to find inspiration: look for online videos to learn new yoga poses or sequences, or read an inspiring article from yoga and mindfulness teachers.

Hopefully, by now you have directly experienced how yoga can benefit your overall wellness. What's important to remember is that yoga is an ongoing practice, and   there will be days when it feels easier than others to practice yoga, but as long as you stay present and dedicated, you will see how much it can change your health for the better.

REFERENCES

American Heart Association. "American Heart Association Recommendations for Physical Activity in Adults and Kids."

Bond Brill, J., et al. "Dose-Response Effect of Walking Exercise on Weight Loss. How Much is Enough?" International Journal of Obesity and Related Metabolic Disorders: Journal of the International Association for the Study of Obesity. 26.11 (2002): 1484–1493. https://doi.org/10.1038/sj.ijo.0802133

Centers for Disease Control and Prevention. "Healthy Eating for a Healthy Weight." U.S. Department of Health and Human Services."

Isath, A., et al. "The Effect of Yoga on Cardiovascular Disease Risk Factors: A Meta-Analysis." Current Problems in Cardiology. 48.5 (2023): 101593. https://doi.org/10.1016/j.cpcardiol.2023.101593

Jayawardena, R., et al. "Exploring the Therapeutic Benefits of Pranayama (Yogic Breathing): A Systematic Review." International Journal of Yoga. 13.2 (2020): 99–110. https://doi.org/10.4103/ijoy.IJOY_37_19

Lauche, R., et al. A Systematic Review and Meta-Analysis on the Effects of Yoga on Weight-Related Outcomes. Preventive Medicine. 87 (2016): 213–232. https://doi.org/10.1016/j.ypmed.2016.03.013

La Greca, S., et al. "Acute and Chronic Effects of Supervised Flexibility Training in Older Adults: A Comparison of Two Different Conditioning Programs." International Journal of Environmental Research and Public Health. 19.24 (2022): 16974. https://doi.org/10.3390/ijerph192416974

McGowan, C. J., et al. "Warm-Up Strategies for Sport and Exercise: Mechanisms and Applications." Sports Medicine. 45.11 (2015): 1523–1546. https://doi.org/10.1007/s40279-015-0376-x

National Center for Complementary and Integrative Health. "Meditation and Mindfulness: What You Need to Know."

National Health Service. "Understanding Calories."

Richardson, C. R., et al. "A Meta-Analysis of Pedometer-Based Walking Interventions and Weight Loss." Annals of Family Medicine. 6.1 (2008): 69–77. https://doi.org/10.1370/afm.761

Sherrington, C., et al. "Exercise for Preventing Falls in Older People Living in the Community." The Cochrane Database of Systematic Reviews. 1.1 (2019): CD012424. https://doi.org/10.1002/14651858.CD012424.pub2

Shin S. "Meta-Analysis of the Effect of Yoga Practice on Physical Fitness in the Elderly." International Journal of Environmental Research and Public Health. 18.21 (2021): 11663. https://doi.org/10.3390/ijerph182111663

Sivaramakrishnan, D., et al. "The Effects of Yoga Compared to Active and Inactive Controls on Physical Function and Health Related Quality of Life in Older Adults—Systematic Review and Meta-Analysis of Randomised Controlled Trials." The International Journal of Behavioral Nutrition and Physical Activity, 16.1 (2019): 33. https://doi.org/10.1186/s12966-019-0789-2

Unick, J. L., et al. "A Preliminary Investigation of Yoga as an Intervention Approach for Improving Long-Term Weight Loss: A Randomized Trial." PLoS ONE. 17.2 (2022): e0263405. https://doi.org/10.1371/journal.pone.0263405

Volpi, E., Nazemi, R., and Fujita, S. "Muscle Tissue Changes with Aging." Current Opinion in Clinical Nutrition and Metabolic Care. 7.4 (2004): 405–410. https://doi.org/10.1097/01.mco.0000134362.76653.b2

Walston J. D. "Sarcopenia in Older Adults." Current Owpinion in Rheumatology. 24.6 (2012): 623–627. https://doi.org/10.1097/BOR.0b013e328358d59b

Woods, K., Bishop, P., & Jones, E. (2007). "Warm-up and Stretching in the Prevention of Muscular Injury." Sports Medicine. 37.12 (2007): 1089–1099. https://doi.org/10.2165/00007256-200737120-00006

World Health Organization. "Cardiovascular Diseases."

BONUS THANK YOU

Thank you for choosing **Chair Yoga for Seniors Over 60**. We hope this book has provided you with the guidance and inspiration needed for your wellness journey. Your commitment to improving your health and well-being is truly commendable. Remember, every small step you take brings you closer to a healthier, happier you. Keep going, and stay motivated!

Don't forget to claim your bonus. Go to your internet browser and type in **https://www.getmovefit.com/chairyogaforseniors** to register for the unlimited and free portal access. There are no hidden extra costs, this is completely free with the purchase of this book.

SCAN ME

The PIN code to unlock your bonus is **11233**

These bonuses are **FREE** and designed to **help you achieve your goals**.

With gratitude,
Linette Cunley

www.ingramcontent.com/pod-product-compliance
Lightning Source LLC
Chambersburg PA
CBHW080850300326

41935CB00042B/1699